Managing the Menopause

About the authors

Dr Sally Hope is a GP, an honorary research fellow at the University of Oxford and a member of the British Menopause Society (BMS).

Margaret Rees is an honorary consultant, a Reader in Women's Health at the University of Oxford and the editor of the Journal of the BMS.

Acknowledgements

The authors and publishers would like to thank Rosalind Grant, author of *Which? Medicine*, for writing Chapter 5 (Hormone replacement therapy) and Janet Brockie, a menopause nurse specialist and a member of the BMS, for writing Chapters 6 (Alternatives to HRT) and 7 (Staying healthy).

Helen Barnett, author of *The Which? Guide to Complementary Therapies*, Sue Davies and Sue Freeman read and commented on the manuscript.

The authors are grateful to Joan Ackrill for her help and typing, and Cathy O'Neil and Wendy Hirsh for their encouragement.

Managing the Menopause

Dr Sally Hope and Margaret Rees

CONSUMERS' ASSOCIATION

Which? Books are commissioned by
Consumers' Association and published by
Which? Ltd, 2 Marylebone Road, London NW1 4DF
Email: books@which.net

Distributed by The Penguin Group:
Penguin Books Ltd, 80 Strand, London WC2R 0RL

First edition August 2004

British Library Cataloguing in Publication Data
A catalogue record for *Managing the Menopause* is available from the British
Library

ISBN 0 85202 9772

For a full list of Which? books, please call 0800 252100, access our website
at www.which.net, or write to Which? Books, Freepost, PO Box 44,
Hertford SG14 1SH

Editorial and production: Joanna Bregosz, Alethea Doran, Nithya Rae,
Barbara Toft
Index: Marie Lorimer
Original cover concept by Sarah Harmer
Cover photograph by Clarissa Leahy/gettyimages

Typeset by Saxon Graphics Ltd, Derby
Printed and bound by Creative Print & Design, Wales

Contents

*An asterisk against the name of an organisation in the text indicates that the address can be found in this section.

Introduction

The menopause is a natural milestone in our lives. It throws up a large number of lifestyle choices which women and their partners need to understand and consider, including contraception and sexual health.

A vast sea change has occurred in the last decade in how women seek information about the menopause. In the early 1990s only 30 per cent of women consulted their doctor or primary care nurse about the menopause. By the late 1990s over 75 per cent had sought information from their family doctor about menopausal issues. *Managing the Menopause* is a distillation of many hundreds of consultations the authors have had with women, and incorporates the facts that most people want to know. The menopause affects the entire family, and often partners and children wish to help and understand the changes that are going on mentally and physically at this time. This book sets out to explain them for the woman concerned and all those close to her.

The vast majority of women in the UK do not take hormone replacement therapy (HRT), but they want to know about the benefits and risks of taking medicines to help them through their menopause in order to make their own informed, evidence-based choice. The whole field of HRT and the menopause is continually changing as more medical studies are published. Two huge recent medical trials, the Million Women Study from the UK, and the Women's Health Initiative study from the USA, have given us a lot more, somewhat-conflicting, data. This book presents the data from these trials so women can understand the current controversies in this field of research, and come to their own decision.

Many women use complementary therapies to help relieve menopausal symptoms. Chapter 6 examines the therapies considered most relevant, and also discusses other, natural, ways of managing the menopause. The next chapter looks at a more holistic approach to good health, from which every family member could benefit.

As women age, they are more likely to suffer from disorders such as osteoporosis and heart disease. There are a number of steps they can take to lower the risks of getting these – and other – illnesses. Some chapters in this book are devoted to telling you what you can do to help yourself, and also what the treatment is likely to be if you are diagnosed with some of the more common conditions that affect women of menopausal age.

This book aims to demystify the medical terms used – with the inclusion of chapters on basic physiology and a glossary – and arm you with enough information for you to be able to discuss issues with your GP or nurse and feel in control throughout your menopause.

Chapter 1

The menstrual cycle

Over the last hundred or so years the number of women who live well past the menopause has risen sharply. At present women in the UK can expect to live till 83 years of age, so most will have at least 30 years of postmenopausal life. Indeed, some women are now living longer postmenopausally then premenopausally.

It is interesting to note that while the age of puberty has come down over the years to 11 years, the average age for the onset of the menopause has remained almost constant, at around 51 years.

This chapter looks at the menstrual cycle and the way it changes, from puberty to the start of the menopause.

Puberty

At puberty, major internal biochemical changes manifest themselves in external physical alterations such as breast development. Some of the chemicals responsible are hormones, which are released from the pituitary gland situated in the brain. The hypothalamus in the brain regulates the amount of hormones the pituitary gland releases. The two key hormones are follicle-stimulating hormone (FSH) and luteinising hormone (LH), collectively known as gonadotrophins. These are the stimulating hormones that encourage the ovaries to produce two further hormones, oestrogen and progesterone.

Puberty begins when oestrogen floods into the bloodstream, causing early budding of breast tissue, influencing the development of fat deposits and smoothing the body contours to produce the characteristic female outline. Pubic and underarm hair begins to grow, and special sweat glands, the apocrine glands, located at the entrance to the vagina and anus, under the arms and around the nipples and navel, start to function. While ordinary sweat glands exude an odourless combination of sweat, water and lactic acid, the apocrine glands exude a milky liquid with a characteristic odour. Oestrogen also causes enlargement of the ovaries, from the size of a grape to that of a walnut, which takes 12–24 months following the onset of puberty. The ovaries are then ready for egg production.

Under the influence of FSH and LH from the pituitary gland the first menstruation, or 'menarche', occurs. This represents a major change: a step from girlhood to womanhood. The time of the menarche varies and seems to be influenced by factors such as race, genes, diet and socio-economic background.

During the first year following the menarche it is normal for only three or four episodes of menstruation (periods) to occur, lasting on average five to seven days. Periods become more regular, settling into the usual monthly cycle, as the teenager gets older.

The normal cycle

The reproductive cycle normally lasts an average of 28 days, though it can range from 25 to 35 days. The duration of the menstrual flow may also change from month to month, lasting from two to eight days. Such a range is perfectly normal. The amount of blood lost in a period can also vary a good deal, from 10–100 ml; the average loss is 35–40 ml. A heavy period, known as menorrhagia, is defined as one in which more than 80ml of blood is lost. The highest blood loss ever measured in one period was 1,600 ml.

The first 14 days of the cycle are known as the proliferative phase, and the last 14 days, from ovulation to the onset of menstruation, the secretory phase (see Figure 1).

Ovulation

Within about two years of puberty the process of ovulation begins. At birth the ovaries of a female baby contain approximately two million immature egg cells, called oöcytes. By the menarche only some 300,000 remain, the others having been lost over the years through natural attrition (atresia). A minimum of 1,000 egg cells is thought to be required for the maintenance of the menstrual cycle. At the menarche FSH causes egg cells to mature, usually one at a time. Each egg cell is situated in a follicle in the ovary. The ovarian follicles are lined with granulosa cells, and it is these cells that produce the hormone oestrogen, which, when released into the

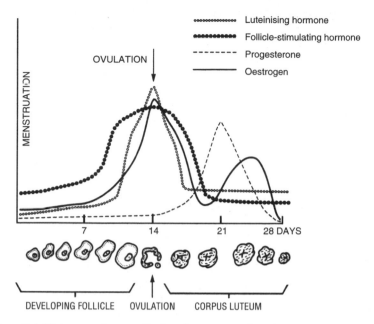

Figure 1 Hormone changes during the menstrual cycle

bloodstream, has a powerful effect on the endometrium, which is the lining of the uterus (womb). The lining thickens and becomes rich in blood vessels: this is the proliferative phase. The ripening egg cell meanwhile pushes its way to the surface of the ovary, where it produces a cyst or blister which ruptures, releasing the egg into the Fallopian tube. Ovulation has then taken place.

This event is caused by a surge in the amount of LH from the pituitary gland. The granulosa cells of the ovarian follicle produce, in addition to oestrogen, a protein-like substance called inhibin. The rising level of inhibin in the bloodstream reduces the amount of FSH secretion from the pituitary, and this in turn initiates the LH surge which induces ovulation.

At the burst follicle, granulosa cells accumulate and fold inwards upon themselves, to form a yellow-pink structure (corpus luteum) on the surface of the ovary. This is the source of the second ovarian hormone, progesterone. Progesterone causes the new tissue of the endometrium, which was laid down under the direction of oestrogen during the proliferative phase, to become softer and sponge-like (secretory phase), ready to receive a fertilised egg.

Fimbriae of Fallopian tube   Ripening follicle

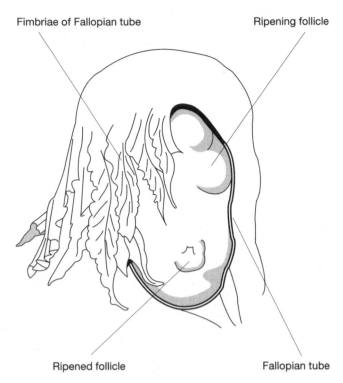

Ripened follicle   Fallopian tube

Figure 2   The ovary and the follicle

The walls of the vagina are kept moist by mucus-producing cells in the neck of the uterus (cervix). During the proliferative phase, the oestrogen produced by the ovary causes the mucus to be thin, watery and clear, assisting the passage of any sperm towards the Fallopian tubes leading from the uterus. In the secretory phase, after ovulation, the progesterone produced from the corpus luteum causes the vaginal mucus to thicken and become more sticky or tenacious. This altered mucus hinders further sperm from entering the Fallopian tubes. Both oestrogen and progesterone tend to cause wave-like contractions in the tubes, assisting the egg in its average six-and-a-half-day journey to the uterus.

If a sperm and egg unite, conception takes place and the fertilised egg (ovum) then travels to the uterus, where it embeds itself in the soft endometrial layer. The delicate communication system that links the hypothalamus, pituitary, ovary and uterus is now activated, with the result that the level of progesterone is increased, and maintained, to ensure the health of the endometrium. Continued progesterone production by the ovary is assured with the formation of a corpus luteum cyst at, or near, the site of the ruptured ovarian follicle. After about the ninth week of pregnancy, the progesterone produced from this cyst is topped up by additional progesterone production from the developing placenta. This nourishing/receiving pad at the end of the umbilical cord delivers nourishment to the foetus.

Research indicates that an adequate blood level of the hormone prolactin is necessary for normal corpus luteal function, further progesterone production, and the maintenance of a healthy pregnancy. Exactly how prolactin influences the normal menstrual cycle is as yet unclear, but it is known that the hypothalamus regulates its production, and release, by the pituitary gland.

Menstruation

If conception does not take place, the ovary continues to produce progesterone and oestrogen until approximately the 24th day of the cycle. At this point the communication mechanism is again activated by the falling oestrogen and progesterone levels. The hypothalamus reduces its controlling releasing hormone to the pituitary gland, which in turn decreases the supply of FSH and LH to the ovary. Consequently, during the last three days of the cycle there is a dramatic reduction in both oestrogen and progesterone, which causes a decrease in blood flow to the uterus. Cell destruction results, and the unnourished uterine lining is shed. The menstrual flow begins as the unwanted endometrium is discarded.

Menstruation is often accompanied by cramps – contractions of the muscle wall of the uterus as it squeezes the endometrium free and assists in its expulsion. Endometrial cells release hormone-like substances called prostaglandins. These have been shown to be of immense importance in the overall balance mechanism of the body.

The perimenopausal cycle

During the fertile years there is a gradual depletion of ovarian follicles, and hence the egg cells they contain. The loss of egg cells accelerates once the number has fallen below 25,000 (usually around the age of 35).

The reason for this acceleration may be genetic (Turner's Syndrome) or age-related; it can also be caused by radiation treatment, chemotherapy, disease or toxins (mumps oöphoritis and cigarette-smoking), or by surgery (see 'Causes of early menopause', below).

At the menopause only a few eggs remain. With the depletion of the follicles, the level of fertility is reduced and oestrogen deficiency begins. As the number of granulosa cells in the follicles reduces, inhibin production also decreases, very gradually. The level of FSH therefore changes little.

By the time a woman is in her early forties the number of granulosa cells decreases to such a degree that the level of inhibin they secrete falls to a critical point; the level of FSH now rises. Although the menstrual periods may still be completely regular and no menopausal symptoms are being experienced, the rising FSH level represents the beginning of the perimenopause.

As follicle depletion continues over the next few years the level of FSH fluctuates, and the menstrual cycle becomes irregular. The amount of menstrual flow also alters, being sometimes lighter and sometimes heavier. FSH levels increase with continuing fluctuations, but there is a marked variation between individual women. Oestrogen production usually remains near-normal in the early years of the perimenopause, therefore symptoms associated with oestrogen deficiency, such as hot flushes (known as hot flashes in American literature) and vaginal dryness, will not yet be evident. As oestrogen levels fall over the next few years the occasional hot flush, increasing tiredness and perhaps dizziness will occur, and menstrual periods may become more irregular with episodes of heavy bleeding.

The menopause

The menopause has been reached when there has been no bleeding for 12 months. This indicates that there is no longer any stimulation of the endometrium by oestrogen and progesterone, but it does not mean that the body is not producing any oestrogen – it is still produced (in small quantities) by the postmenopausal ovaries and from the adrenal glands, which are situated on top of each kidney. Another source of oestrogen is androstenedione, a weak

Definitions

The menopause The medical definition of the menopause is not having a period for 12 months without any other reason for this (see 'Other causes of sudden amenorrhoea', on page 18). If periods still occur, however irregularly, the menopause has not taken place.

Pre-menopause This term can mean the whole of a woman's reproductive life before the menopause, or the few years just before the menopause.

Perimenopause In the two to three years before periods actually stop forever, a woman tends to notice symptoms such as hot flushes and irregular periods. This is called the perimenopause. It is a time when the hormones are beginning to change and 'hormonal chaos' occurs.

Postmenopause This is any time after the woman's final menstrual period. Because of the definition of the menopause, women do not know they are in the postmenopausal phase until a year after their last period.

Menopausal transition This is another term for the perimenopause before the final menstrual period, but when women are experiencing symptoms.

Premature menopause The average age for periods to stop is between 49 and 51. There is a huge variation of the menopause in different women, and any age between 45 and 54 is considered to be within normal limits. The menopause is early, or premature, if it happens before the age of 45 (see 'Causes of early menopause', on pages 16–17).

Induced menopause This is an abnormal early menopause brought about either by direct surgery (for example, when the ovaries are removed) or from damage during other pelvic surgery (for example, when a hysterectomy is carried out, even though the intention was to preserve the ovaries).

androgen steroid which is converted in the liver, and in fat tissue, to a weak form of oestrogen called oestrone. However, oestrone production rarely reaches sufficient quantity to prevent menopausal symptoms and signs (see Chapter 2).

The menopause tends to take place between the ages of 45 and 54, and especially between 49 and 51. It is likely to happen about two years earlier in cigarette-smokers and in women who have had a hysterectomy (removal of the uterus) without removal of both ovaries (see 'Causes of early menopause', below).

Causes of early menopause

A few women cease to menstruate in their thirties. The egg cells within the ovaries disappear spontaneously, causing sudden cessation of menstruation and abrupt hormonal changes. If the ovaries fail before the age of 45 it is known as a premature menopause. This can be caused by natural factors (primary premature ovarian failure) or medical treatment (secondary ovarian failure).

Primary premature ovarian failure

In the vast majority of women the cause of an early menopause is unknown. Quite often it runs in families, so if you are concerned that you might be starting your menopause early, try to find out at what age your mother and grandmother started theirs.

Early menopause can, very rarely, be caused by diseases of the immune system which can also be associated with diabetes and an inactive thyroid or poor functioning of the adrenal glands. It could also be caused by abnormal chromosomes – for example, in women with Down's Syndrome or Turner's Syndrome. Abnormal hormone production or hormone receptors may also result in early menopause. There are some other very rare causes of a premature menopause. If your periods have stopped (known medically as amenorrhoea) for no obvious reason before you turn 45 (see 'Other causes of sudden amenorrhoea', on page 18) you should consult your doctor.

The ovarian hormones

The two significant female ovarian hormones, oestrogen and progesterone, have a profound effect on the body. During the perimenopause, and at the menopause, the changes that take place are caused in particular by falling levels of these two hormones.

Oestrogen

Oestrogen attaches itself to the surface of cells and in organs where it is needed, influencing the functioning of that organ either by its

---

Secondary premature ovarian failure

The most common cause for ovarian failure is the surgical removal of ovaries (known medically as bilateral oöphorectomy).

Before a woman has a hysterectomy (surgical removal of the uterus), the surgeon usually goes through the pros and cons of whether the ovaries should be conserved (left intact), depending on the reason for the hysterectomy. If the ovaries have been conserved at hysterectomy, they should continue to produce natural oestrogen and progesterone after the operation. However, there is good evidence that some women who have had a hysterectomy with conservation of the ovaries still experience an early menopause because the blood supply to the ovaries was compromised at surgery. This is a well-known complication of a hysterectomy and, prior to surgery, must be understood as a possible outcome.

One of the problems of a hysterectomy is the loss of the natural marker of ovarian function: periods. Some women who have a hysterectomy do not have any symptoms of the menopause but are found biochemically to have gone through the 'change' without symptoms. Sometimes, in young women who have had a hysterectomy with ovarian conservation, a premature menopause is missed because it can masquerade as many other non-specific symptoms, such as general tiredness and depression. It is advisable that any woman under the age of 45 who has a hysterectomy with ovarian conservation should have a blood test once a year to check hormone levels.

Infections such tuberculosis and mumps are extremely rare causes of ovarian failure.

Other causes of sudden amenorrhoea

Menopause is not the only reason for the cessation of periods. Other causes include:

- pregnancy or breastfeeding
- hormonal contraception
- extreme weight loss or anorexia nervosa
- overactive thyroid
- polycystic ovaries
- extreme stress
- travel though different time zones
- hormonal imbalances.

presence (during the fertile years) or by its absence (after the menopause). The chief source of oestrogen is the granulosa cells.

What does oestrogen do?

Oestrogen

- maintains the health and proper functioning of the genital organs
- causes the endometrium (uterus lining) to thicken in the proliferative phase of the menstrual cycle
- softens the cervix and produces the thin mucus in which the sperm can swim
- enhances the chance of fertilisation by improving the mobility of the egg as it passes down the Fallopian tubes
- acts with inhibin to affect the hypothalamus in its regulation of the menstrual cycle
- acts to maintain the health of the walls of blood vessels
- maintains supply of collagen to the skin, which promotes skin elasticity, and calcium to the bones, which keeps them strong
- influences the development of the breasts and maintains breast structure and the milk ducts
- affects the thickness of the skin and the condition of the hair
- causes the emergence of typical female shape and form at puberty.

Progesterone

The second female hormone produced by the ovary is progesterone, which is broken down by the liver and secreted in the urine as pregnanediol. Synthetic progesterone (progestogen) is used with natural oestrogens for the control of menopausal symptoms.

What does progesterone do?

Progesterone

- transforms the proliferative endometrium to the secretory form in the second half of the menstrual cycle
- changes the cervical mucus in the second half of the menstrual cycle from a thin and watery substance to one which is thicker and tenacious
- tends to reduce the acidity level of the vagina
- joins with oestrogen to lower the levels of FSH and LH by acting with inhibin on the hypothalamus
- raises the basal body temperature, which can be measured at the time of ovulation
- maintains pregnancy through an intricate hormonal interaction
- stimulates development of breast tissue, particularly the alveoli gland system
- encourages water and salt retention (although less so than synthetic progestogen)
- enhances the immune system through intricate links with prostaglandins and immunoglobulins
- may influence mood during the latter half of the menstrual cycle.

Premenstrual syndrome

Premenstrual syndrome (PMS) is a complex disorder for which commonly reported symptoms include fatigue, headache, backache, aggression, depression, irritability, mood swings, weight gain, skin eruptions, food craving, feelings of bloatedness and sore breasts. It is not unusual for PMS to worsen slightly in the perimenopause.

Relaxation techniques for stress management, exercise and changes to the diet often help women with mild symptoms to cope.

Although it is often thought that PMS is caused by fluctuations in the levels of oestrogen and progesterone, this is not necessarily the case. It is interesting to note that oestrogen and progesterone levels are similar when measured in PMS sufferers and 'controls', and further research needs to be done in this complex and difficult field.

Testosterone

This primary male hormone is produced in small quantities in women by both the ovaries and the adrenal glands. If too much is produced it may cause masculinisation and give rise to an excess of unwanted hair (hirsutism).

In postmenopausal women the ovary tends to produce more testosterone than in pre-menopausal years, and this may explain why older women tend to show a degree of defeminisation and hirsutism.

The postmenopausal ovary is hormonally active for several years after the menopause. One function is to produce a small indirect amount of oestrogen (estradiol) from testosterone by a chemical process called aromatisation. The oestrogen thus produced may help to protect the vagina and parts of the urethra from early thinning or atrophy.

Chapter 2

Symptoms and signs of the menopause

In medical terms, the menopause is considered to have occurred after a woman has not had any periods for 12 months. However, often women have menopausal symptoms, such as hot flushes, for two to three years before their periods finally cease (i.e. in the peri-menopause) and for many years after. Those women who do not have periods – either because they take hormonal forms of contraception which stop them having periods, or because they have had a hysterectomy with ovarian conservation – have lost the external 'marker' of their cycle so may not know whether they have reached the menopause or not, although other symptoms can give them an indication.

About 20 to 30 per cent of women do not experience any symptoms associated with the menopause. There is enormous variation, both within a community and across different ethnic groups, as well as in the same ethnic group in different parts of the world. This has caused much interest in the extent to which diet and lifestyle may account for the differences in how women feel as they go through the menopause. For example, Japanese women report fewer symptoms than American women. Some have argued that this is a cultural difference, but others have pointed to the traditional Japanese diet of soya beans, which are high in phytoestrogens (see Chapter 10). Much research is being done in this area at present. Other factors also play a part: for example, a Swedish study showed that women with a higher education who also exercised regularly were more likely to be symptom-free than less well-educated women or those who did not exercise regularly. The interaction of education, lifestyle and expectations, relating to how women feel about their bodies at the time of the menopause and what symptoms they can tolerate, is a very complex issue.

Summary of the symptoms and signs of the menopause

Symptoms

- periods irregular, for up to four years, and then stop
- hot flushes and sweats
- changes to skin and hair
- memory changes
- changes in sexuality
- changes in emotion

Long-term problems

- recurrent urinary infections
- vaginal dryness
- osteoporosis
- cardiovascular disease
- Alzheimer's disease.

Although the terms 'symptoms' and 'signs' are often used interchangeably, strictly speaking a symptom is a complaint of which the patient is herself aware, such as hot flushes. A sign is determined by medical examination: for example, raised blood pressure or an altered cholesterol level.

As ovarian follicles become fewer in number so the amount of circulating 17β-oestradiol (the isolated form of oestrogen produced by the granulosa cells) falls, and symptoms of oestrogen deficiency become more evident. In overweight women, however, such symptoms are lessened (although not prevented) by the presence of oestrone, a weaker form of oestrogen which is produced by conversion of a weak androgen steroid called androstenedione in fatty tissues.

Oestrogen deficiency is linked with, but not always entirely responsible for, the various symptoms and signs which occur around the menopause. These may be considered as physical, psychological or sexual.

Physical symptoms

Changes in menstrual flow

During the perimenopause, menstrual flow may alter in both volume and duration. Changes in the length of bleeding and the length of the cycle happen in women after the age of 40. Often the first sign is that the cycle changes and actually shortens. Such alterations indicate changes taking place in the control mechanism between the hypothalamus and the pituitary gland (see Chapter 1).

Erratic and irregular menstrual bleeding – known as dysfunctional uterine bleeding – is often heavy and may require medical attention to bring it under control. Simple medication is usually sufficient, but possible causes other than the menopause have first to be ruled out, perhaps by exploratory procedures such as ultrasound examination, endometrial biopsy or dilatation and curettage (see Chapter 9), as well as by blood tests. Such possible causes include polyps or fibroids. Fibroids are benign thickenings of the muscle of the wall of the uterus. When the uterus contracts during a period to try to reduce the bleeding, the fibroids get in the way and stop the efficient shut-down of the bleeding points, which can lead to very heavy periods. Polyps are outgrowths either of the cervix or the inside of the uterus. Polyps and fibroids can be found either by physical examination, because the uterus is slightly larger than would be expected, or by an ultrasound examination.

Very rarely, dysfunctional bleeding can be a sign of an abnormal thickening of the lining of the uterus that could eventually lead to uterine cancer. Uterine cancer is extremely rare in women under 50. See Chapter 8 for more about this.

While irregular periods are quite normal, irregular bleeding – any bleeding that occurs between periods, after intercourse or after the menopause – is not, and should be investigated. Again, this may be a sign of a polyp or irregular thickening of the lining of the uterus, or of uterine cancer. About one in ten women who present with post-menopausal bleeding has uterine cancer. This type of cancer has a very good chance of being cured, if surgery is done quickly, as the cancer is contained in the muscular uterus and spreads only after a long time.

A common cause of postmenopausal bleeding from the vagina itself is atrophic vaginitis – see 'Genital and urinary changes', below.

Pain associated with normal or abnormal menstrual bleeding is known as dysmenorrhoea. It may be caused by infection, fibroids, endometriosis or prostaglandin imbalance (see Chapter 8).It is rare for periods to become more painful as a result of perimenopausal changes, but if they do this should be investigated.

Genital and urinary changes

Oestrogen has a local effect on the vagina, to keep secretions active, so that the area is moist and elastic. Because oestrogen levels drop after the menopause, the lining of the vagina weakens and thins, its blood supply diminishes, and it becomes drier. Some women experience soreness and discomfort with sexual intercourse, or even at other times. The walls of the vagina can become so dry that tiny bleeding points occur. This is known as atrophic vaginitis, and can be treated with local oestrogen creams or pessaries. Because this treatment is local, so the oestrogen is not absorbed into the body, the risks of full hormone replacement therapy (see Chapter 5) are not incurred.

The bladder and urethra (the tube leading from the bladder to the outside of the body) are also affected. The lining shrinks, becomes thinner and drier, and is more likely to crack and split. This also makes it more vulnerable to infection. Again, local oestrogen treatment can help postmenopausal women troubled by recurrent urinary infections.

The trigone bladder (doorway to the urethra) also atrophies, leading to a pressing need to pass urine, and to pass it frequently. Sometimes incontinence occurs after sneezing or coughing. Urge incontinence – an involuntary loss of urine which may occur with the sudden urge to urinate – responds well to pelvic floor exercises (see Chapter 8). These exercises, taught to women after they have had a baby, can help to improve the tone of the pelvic floor. Stress incontinence – involuntary loss of a little urine on coughing, sneezing or laughing – may require surgical correction (see Chapter 8).

Skin and hair changes

At the perimenopause an increasing dryness and thinning of the skin, brittle nails and changes to the hair may be noticed. Thirty per

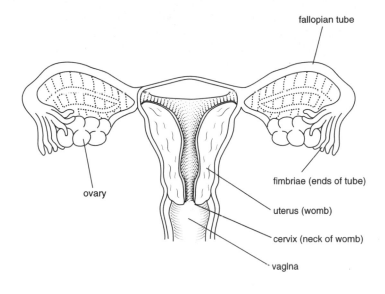

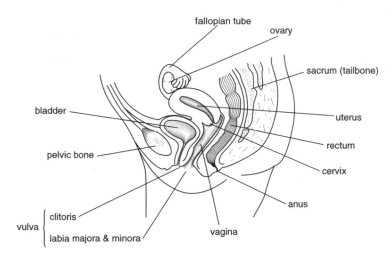

Figure 1   Female reproductive system

cent of skin collagen, which forms a large part of the connective
support tissue of the skin, is lost in the first ten years after the
menopause. This causes further thinning of the skin, which
increases the incidence of bruising and gives a transparent, waxy
appearance, and loss of skin tone, i.e. wrinkles. Hair roots originate

from the deep layers of skin connective tissue and are therefore affected by lack of oestrogen. All of these symptoms are caused by lack of water in the tissue combined with reduced blood supply. Hormone replacement therapy (HRT) has been shown to restore lost collagen to pre-menopausal levels within six months, due in part to the fact that there are oestrogen receptors in the connective tissue. It increases the water content of the skin as well as improving its blood flow.

The actual growth of hair depends more on male hormones than oestrogen, which mainly affects the distribution of hair. As oestrogen levels fall, male hormones (androgens) increase, stimulating hair growth on the upper body and face. Glandular function also often becomes less efficient, giving rise to dryness of the throat and burning of the eyes and mouth; bowel upsets and constipation may also occur.

Vasomotor symptoms (hot flushes, sweats and palpitations)

The most common menopausal symptoms, experienced to some degree by 80 per cent of women, are vasomotor ones – hot flushes, night sweats and palpitations. The exact cause of a hot flush is unknown, but there is a probable link with breakdown in temperature control by the hypothalamus as oestrogen production declines during the perimenopause. This in turn influences the sympathetic nervous system, which dilates the blood vessels and gives rise to an increased heart rate (palpitations) and sometimes headaches. Brain chemicals called catecholamines and opiate-like substances are also thought to influence the heat regulatory mechanism. It is interesting to note that men treated with anti-testosterone drugs for prostate cancer also experience serious hot flushes – they are not unique to the female.

Vasomotor symptoms are most noticeable just before and at the menopause – studies show that 40 to 80 per cent of women experience hot flushes within the two-year timespan surrounding their final menstrual period. Symptoms continue for more than a year in most women and for longer than five years in 29 to 50 per cent. But, unlike other menopausal complaints, vasomotor symptoms decrease and disappear as hormone levels stabilise (although some women still experience hot flushes for many years later).

Hot flushes usually start as a pressure sensation in the head, followed by a feeling of heat which may extend from the head to the neck, upper chest and back, then spread to the whole body. They can occur at any time of the day or night. Night-time flushes and sweats are particularly troublesome because they disturb sleep, leading to extreme tiredness and irritability, and may also disturb a partner's sleep, putting a strain on relationships. Some women can have over 100 hot flushes a day, while others only have a few occasionally at night.

HRT (see Chapter 5) helps to control the hormone level fluctuations, usually easing vasomotor symptoms within a week of starting treatment, although it may be two or three months before the full benefits are felt. Non-hormonal approaches are reviewed in Chapter 6.

Breast changes

The breasts develop at puberty under the influence of oestrogen. Around the menopause some gradual change may be apparent, owing to the reduction of both oestrogen and progesterone. The breasts may become smaller, with the nipples also reducing and becoming flatter and the areola darkening slightly; there may be some roughness and thinning of the skin.

Bone and cardiovascular changes

Both bone and blood vessels undergo change at and after the menopause. Bone mass reduces more rapidly than during the perimenopause, and heart disease in particular is more likely to develop. These problems are considered at greater length in Chapters 3 and 4.

Psychological symptoms

Emotional changes are commonly complained of by women experiencing the menopause. These include mood swings, irritability, anxiety, a poor memory, lack of concentration, loss of energy, tiredness and depression.

It is likely that these psychological symptoms at this stage in life are caused at least in part by a lack of oestrogen. But to what extent they also result from, or are exacerbated by, other menopausal

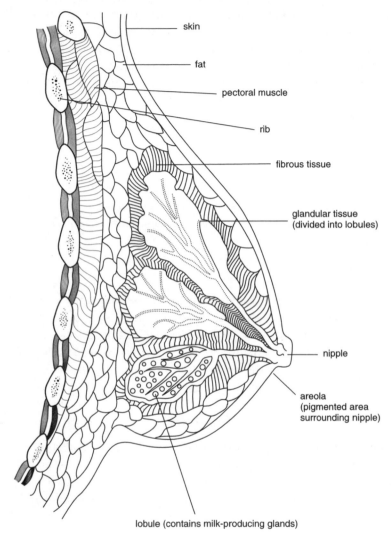

skin

fat

pectoral muscle

rib

fibrous tissue

glandular tissue
(divided into lobules)

nipple

areola
(pigmented area
surrounding nipple)

lobule (contains milk-producing glands)

Figure 2 Structure of the breast

symptoms is hard to say and will vary between individuals. For example, loss of sleep caused by hot flushes and night-time wakefulness is likely to give rise to fatigue, irritability and other alterations in normal functioning. Some research suggests that oestrogen exerts a direct effect that helps to counteract irritability, fatigue, insomnia, anxiety and depression, and it is certainly true that, in their pre-menopausal adult lives, most women experience a mild change in their mood over their monthly cycle. Usually they feel positive and energetic when their oestrogen levels are high but, towards the end of the cycle when the oestrogen drops and the progesterone rises, they begin to feel grumpy, bloated and snappy: a collection of symptoms more commonly known as premenstrual syndrome (see Chapter 1).

It could be argued that for many women the menopause is the most stressful time in their lives. They may be caring for elderly and frail relatives or facing the death of a parent or loved one; they may have teenage children in their 'rebellious years' and a partner who is going through a mid-life crisis. It is often the woman who bears the brunt of providing emotional support, with little energy left for herself.

Social factors also play a part. Research has shown that women of lower socio-economic groups have more psychological menopausal problems than those who are educated and financially secure, with pleasant homes, regular holidays and, possibly, rewarding jobs and/or sympathetic partners. A woman who is tired and over-worked, with little understanding of health matters and limited access to information, may well have more difficulties in coming to terms with menopausal change. Similarly, a woman without children, who has not had to experience the 'empty nest' syndrome of offspring leaving home, may exhibit fewer psychological symptoms during the menopause. But there is no set pattern and the subject is a complex one.

Depression

From puberty onwards, women suffer from depression and anxiety disorders two to three times more often than do men. At times of marked hormonal change – premenstrually, postnatally and around the menopause – this tendency to depression is heightened. It is quite probable that the fluctuating balance between oestrogen and progesterone at these times influences the intricate web of chemical messengers in the brain, which in turn initiates the psychological symptoms, in particular depression, to which some women are particularly susceptible.

When referring to depression, however, it is important to distinguish between depressed mood and depressive disorder. These are quite different conditions.

Depressed mood refers to low spirits, sadness or despondency, which are common symptoms around the menopause and are considered to be caused by lack of oestrogen. Depressed mood may be a response to hot flushes, sweats or disturbed sleep. HRT may be of assistance, although some studies indicate that it is no better than a placebo. Moreover, even if HRT **does** increase well-being or enhance mood, this does not automatically mean that low levels of oestrogen cause depression. Psychosocial factors are just as likely to be responsible.

Depressive disorder is quite different from 'depressed mood', and is far more serious and more debilitating. A serious depression may have the following symptoms: lack of concentration and interest; loss of appetite, weight and sex drive; feelings of impending doom, guilt and worthlessness; slow and quiet speech; early-morning waking and an inability to take decisions. Depressive disorder is not common at the menopause, and nor have studies revealed any relationship between the menopause and depressive disorder. A depressive disorder is usually treated with antidepressant medication together with cognitive behavioural therapy and/or counselling.

Alzheimer's disease (dementia)

Alzheimer's disease is by far the most common form of dementia in the UK. About 75 per cent of dementia sufferers have Alzheimer's; in the other 25 per cent the condition has vascular causes, resulting from mini-strokes. Alzheimer's is a progressive degenerative brain disease which impairs memory, behaviour and thinking. As nerve cells in the cortex of the brain disappear, sufferers typically show signs of forgetfulness, speech problems, difficulty with daily activities, and geographical disorientation, as well as irritability, sleep disturbance and a tendency to wander. Ultimately, the disorder is fatal. Some 10 per cent of the UK population develop dementia in retirement.

Women are more prone to Alzheimer's than are men. It is more common in thin women than obese women and also in those who have suffered a previous myocardial infarction (heart attack) or hip fracture, both of which (see Chapters 3 and 4) suggest a link with oestrogen deficiency. The age of onset of Alzheimer's disease is later in women who have taken HRT than in those who have never taken it or in those who have gone through a premature menopause. Studies have shown that verbal memory has been maintained, and reaction speed and attention span increased, in women who have received HRT. However, it is possible that in these studies the women who accepted HRT may have been a sub-group whose behaviour patterns would lead them to have a reduced risk of cognitive impairment anyway. It is not known which types of women would benefit most from HRT in this way. Nor is it known what the effective dosage and duration of administration of oestrogen might be to optimise the cognitive benefits and minimise unwanted side-effects. Indeed, the most recent trial of combined oestrogen and progestogen in women over 75 years of age showed an unexpected doubling of the risk of dementia from 1 per cent to 2 per cent, but the significance for younger users still needs to be clarified.

Sexual symptoms

Complex biological, emotional and social factors influence sexual behaviour. Sexual difficulties, which may include poor sexual response, discomfort during intercourse, reduced libido and loss of interest in the sexual partner, are common during the peri-menopausal years.

As described earlier in this chapter, oestrogen, when plentiful, maintains the size, shape, lining and flexibility of the vagina. It also profoundly influences the vagina's response to touch, through its effect on sensation, lubrication and blood supply. Insufficient oestrogen can cause changes that make sexual intercourse uncom-fortable, painful or even impossible. Other effects include difficulty in achieving orgasm – often due to loss in quality of pleasurable genital sensation – and reduced arousal. An understanding partner will appreciate that the vaginal dryness associated with the menopause will take longer to overcome during foreplay (the best method of lubrication yet devised). But if the difficulties are more severe it is well worth discussing them with a doctor so that they can be dealt with at an early stage.

As we have seen, local oestrogen treatments can be very helpful for severe vaginal dryness. They also improve the general tone of the pelvic floor. Simple over-the-counter lubricating jelly is useful in alleviating mild vaginal dryness. However, by no means all women need hormone replacement to maintain good sexual function after the menopause. An active sex life in itself plays a major role in keeping the sexual organs in good condition.

Beyond the age of 50 an increasing proportion of women cease all forms of sexual activity. This is due in part to the fact that half of the women in this age group live alone and may have difficulty finding a partner. Ill-health may reduce sexual interest, as may the side-effects from medications taken for example as treatment for depressive disorders or blood pressure control. Menopausal symptoms such as tiredness, irritability and depression, hot flushes and sleep disturbance can also reduce sexual desire, as can relationship conflicts arising from sexual difficulties. Furthermore, many men over 50 suffer from impotence. This can have many possible causes, including depression, hypertension, carcinoma of the prostate, diabetes mellitus (the cause may be the conditions themselves or some of the medications taken for treatment) or heavy alcohol drinking, but can be effectively treated in some cases by counselling, a change of medication, or self-administered injections to produce erection enhancement. (For more about impotence see *250 Medical Questions Answered*, from Which? Books). Male impotence is sometimes related to the female menopause. In this case it usually stems from fear of hurting the partner, and may be compounded by a lack of arousal in the woman.

In Western society attitudes towards sex have changed greatly over the last few decades. The use of the oral contraceptive pill has been partly responsible, but greater freedom and openness in the discussion of sexual matters have been of equal importance. Today women should expect continuation of a healthy sex life far beyond the menopause. The understanding and communication of problems will help them to achieve, and sustain, a fulfilling sex life.

The menopause across cultures

As indicated at the beginning of this chapter, the menopause experience varies enormously worldwide. Even among different ethnic groups in the same country there are significant differences in symptom reporting. Many of the studies comparing the menopause across different cultures indicate that the majority of women around the world do not find the menopause to be a difficult time. Interest has focused on diet: specifically, on phyto-estrogens (see Chapter 10), which are chemicals found in soya and other beans, which form the staple diet in much of Asia. In Western countries, about 80 per cent of women experience hot flushes and sweats. There is a much lower reporting of these symptoms in women in India, Indonesia, Japan and China, and in rural Mayans living in Yucatan Mexico. Indeed, the reporting of flushes is nonexistent in some non-Western societies.

It is not understood why there is such a difference in this respect between countries and races. It is debatable whether it is due to sociological or cultural differences, such as language and expectations. The association between the hormonal changes and symptoms at the menopause is complex, and is likely to be influenced to by many factors. These may include genetics, biological differences, social environment, physical environment, support networks, children, diet, affluence, frailty, education, attitudes, beliefs, fears and so on.

Although there are unanswered questions, there are, perhaps, lessons to be learned from other cultures. In many non-Western societies, age is revered and associated with wisdom. Consequently, the menopause is welcomed as a positive event, bringing an increase in status. Women in these societies are more likely to view the menopause as a normal part of ageing and not to associate it with illness. Among certain castes in India, for example, the cessation of menstruation signals a woman's emergence from purdah, allowing her to mix freely with the male sex and to counsel younger members of her community. In Sub-Saharan Africa and Ethiopia, post-menopausal women are accorded great respect and special status. (Of course, life expectancy in the developing world is substantially lower than that in industrialised countries, at about 40 to 50 years, and contraception is not practised, so women will have spent much of their lives since puberty either pregnant or giving birth – potentially risky experiences in themselves. Therefore simply to reach the menopause confers status in a way that does not happen in the West, and indeed the last pregnancy may itself mark the point of transition to the menopause.)

In Western culture, in contrast, ageing in general and the menopause in particular tend to be regarded negatively. Our society pursues a cult of youth and universally glorifies the desirability of the younger female at the expense of the mature woman. Faced with images of unattainable youthfulness in the media and society's preference for youth in most other areas of life, including the job market, the prospect of the menopause may seem to the middle-aged woman like a brutal reminder that the 'best' years of her life are now behind her. This raises the possibility that our society, which may be seen to discriminate against the older person and which concentrates on the problems associated with the menopause, may be contributing to a negative attitude, and even to a poor experience of this stage of life.

Dealing with the menopause as a natural life event, rather than a pathological event (which could be said to be the attitude implied by orthodox medicine), might actually improve a woman's experience and reduce the need for treatment. Increasingly, women in the West are coming to view the approach of the menopause as a time for reflection and for reassessment of life's goals. Free from the demands of raising families, for example, it can bring new opportunities and challenges. Putting life into perspective and feeling in control of the change in one's life can often greatly assist the self-management of menopausal symptoms.

Chapter 3

Osteoporosis

Osteoporosis, or 'brittle bone disease', results from low bone density, which makes the bones more susceptible to fracture. It is known as the 'silent epidemic', because people are not aware that they have a low bone density until a low-impact fracture occurs. A low-impact, or 'fragility', fracture is defined as a fracture resulting from a fall from standing height or less. Osteoporosis is of increasing significance for women as they get older, because the bones lose their strength after the menopause. Men also develop osteoporosis, but usually much later than women because they have a higher peak bone mass in their twenties and do not suffer the rapid bone loss that women have in their fifties. The same risk factors and contributory diseases for osteoporosis affect both men and women.

Osteoporosis-related fractures cost the NHS a huge amount of money: over £1.7 billion a year. And, as our life expectancy increases, the burden of osteoporosis on our healthcare system and social services will continue to increase. In the UK there are 50,000 wrist fractures and 60,000 hip fractures each year. Vertebral (spinal) body fractures are thought to number about 40,000 a year, but the actual figure may well be a lot higher. Hip fractures account for 20 per cent of orthopaedic bed occupancy in the UK and are associated with up to a 30-per-cent death rate in the first year after the fracture. A third of women who have had a hip fracture lose their independence subsequently.

Active bones

Many people think that bones are inactive, like stone. This is very far from the truth. Bones have a good blood supply for nutrition, and are constantly 'remodelling' themselves to combat the wear and tear of supporting the weight of the human body over the years. Bone turnover is controlled by two types of cells: **osteoclasts**, which are continually nibbling (reabsorbing) bone to smooth away old bones, and **osteoblasts**, which lay down new bone and strengthen it with calcium. This is how bones can grow from babyhood to adulthood.

Bone structure

Bones are designed to withstand the amount of stress and strain the body imposes on them. Those that will take more stress are denser and more compact. Bone has an outer sheath or membrane, called the **periosteum**, covering the dense outer compact bone: the **cortical** layer. Below this is the spongy, or **trabecular**, layer of bone.

Within the leg and arm bones, which contain little trabecular substance except at their ends, are hollow spaces filled with bone marrow. The wrist bones, the vertebrae and the neck of the femur (the thigh bone) contain trabecular bone but no bone marrow space. Vertebrae have little of the heavy cortical bone, but their cubical shape lends strength to their trabecular composition.

Bone composition and formation

Bone is made up of approximately one-third **collagen**, a protein, (the 'matrix') and two-thirds mineral. Collagen, along with the protein **elastin**, greatly increases the elastic properties of bone and helps to resist stretching forces. The mineral component of bone is mainly calcium, and when this is lost the bone becomes brittle.

Osteoblast cells lay down the matrix and help to deposit calcium, and osteoclast cells, originating from bone marrow, destroy collagen and break down bone. Through a complicated process called 'coupling', osteoclast and osteoblast cells act together to remodel bone. Their action is controlled, negatively and positively, by bone-active hormones and growth factors. These are:

- **parathyroid hormone (PTH)**, which acts on osteoblasts
- **calcitonin**, a hormone that acts on osteoclasts
- **vitamin D**, which acts on osteoclasts and osteoblasts
- **insulin**, a hormone that promotes growth of bone cells
- **oestrogen**, a hormone that acts on osteoblasts.

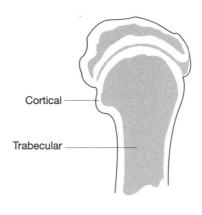

Cortical

Trabecular

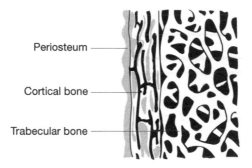

Periosteum

Cortical bone

Trabecular bone

Figure 1 Structure of long bone

Bone density increases during the teenage years and reaches a peak some time in the thirties. This peak bone density is sustained for some years but begins to decline in the mid-forties. For six to ten years after the menopause, women lose bone rapidly. After that, bone loss continues but at a slower rate for the rest of a woman's life. Once the skeleton density drops below a certain level, even minor trauma such as a soft fall or a twisting vigorous turn can cause a fragility fracture.

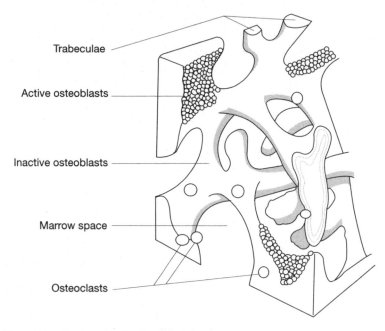

Figure 2 Structure of trabecular bone

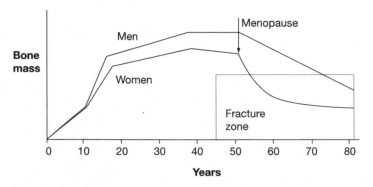

Figure 3 Changes in bone mass with age over years for men and women

Causal and risk factors for osteoporosis

The three main factors that determine whether a woman develops osteoporosis are:

- the **peak bone mass** (how strong the bones are in her mid-twenties and thirties)
- **how fast the bones thin** after the menopause
- the **length of her life** after the menopause.

Genetic elements also play a part. There is a definite pattern in the susceptibility to osteoporosis across different ethnic groups, the risk being highest in Caucasians and lowest in Afro-Caribbean people. There does also seem to be a family history correlation, especially between close female relatives (i.e. mothers or sisters), although male relatives too are relevant.

   Physical characteristics are also significant. Women with a very low body mass index (see Chapter 7 for an explanation of BMI) are at higher risk of osteoporosis. This is because they have no fat tissue to produce extra oestrogen (oestrone, a weaker oestrogen, is produced by conversion of androstenedione, a hormone in fatty tissues – see Chapter 2). Similarly, women who lack oestrogen for any reason, and who are not treated with HRT (see later in this chapter), have a higher rate of osteoporosis. Such reasons include a premature menopause (before the age of 45); an early hysterectomy (before the age of 45), especially if both ovaries are removed; or missing periods for six months or more (for reasons other than pregnancy). Women who have suffered from anorexia nervosa during their twenties, thirties or forties, or those who have had the condition in the past but who are still very thin during this stage of their life, have very low bone densities and are therefore at very high risk of osteoporosis. This includes women with anorexia nervosa who are also compulsive exercisers, because the exercise does not counteract the effect of the extremely low BMI.

   Significant factors that can improve bone density and peak bone mass are:

- a diet rich in **calcium and vitamin D**
- **not smoking**
- taking regular **weight-bearing exercise** (e.g. jogging for 20 minutes, three times a week).

A combination of deficient diet, smoking, and a sedentary way of life is therefore the worst kind of lifestyle in terms of increasing the risk of osteoporosis. A number of other factors, detailed below, also exacerbate the risk. These apply equally to men and to women.

Diet

A high calcium intake during childhood and adolescence improves peak bone mass and, in postmenopausal women, calcium and vitamin D can slow down bone loss. (Vitamin D is necessary in order to absorb calcium effectively.) See the box on page 47 for information on calcium-rich foods – but remember, however, that it is important not to have too much animal protein (such as meat or dairy products), salt or caffeine, because in excessive quantities these can reduce the body's ability to absorb and retain calcium. See Chapter 7 for more about eating for strong bones.

The main source of vitamin D is sunlight – the body makes the vitamin through the action of sunlight on the skin – so even in the winter it is important to go outdoors for walks.

There is some concern that the consumption of large quantities of carbonated drinks can lower bone density because of the displacement of calcium by phosphate in the drinks. It is also not clear whether this is an additive effect, in that if people are drinking fizzy drinks they may drink less milk, and so the diet is less rich in calcium. The stereotypical teenage lifestyle that involves drinking fizzy drinks, sitting all day in front of a computer and smoking, is the worst possible thing for young people's future bone mass.

Smoking

Cigarette smoking is a high risk factor for osteoporosis. This is in part because women who smoke have their menopause one-and-a-half to three years earlier than non-smokers. (Also, cigarette smokers tend to be thinner than people who don't smoke.) Furthermore, the nicotine in tobacco is thought to be toxic to the cells in bone that are responsible for the formation of new bone, so smokers are more likely to have lower bone mass than non-smokers.

Sedentary lifestyle/immobility

Not moving is bad for bones. Immobilisation, even for short periods of a few weeks, results in rapid bone loss. Any housebound or bedbound person must try to do active exercises to prevent osteoporosis. It has been shown that over an 18-month period there is a significant increase in bone mineral density in people undertaking weight-bearing exercise for short periods of time (20 to 30 minutes), three to five times a week. It does have to be weight-bearing exercise, however; swimming, which is relatively weightless, is good for the cardiovascular system but not good for bones. (Interestingly, astronauts who spend periods of time weightless develop rapid, severe osteoporosis.) Even in extreme old age, i.e. for people in their eighties and nineties, exercise can have a positive effect. People who have suffered paralysis for any reason (stroke, spinal injury, head injury or any neurological paralysis) will have osteoporotic bones in the area of the body that is paralysed. Specific exercises and artificial stimulation of the muscles in the paralysed area have been shown to increase bone mineral density.

Exercise also improves muscle strength and balance, reducing the likelihood of falls and fractures.

Heavy alcohol consumption

This is associated with osteoporosis through a combination of factors. Alcohol has a toxic effect on the osteoblast cells, which in heavy drinkers do not work properly to lay down new bone. The fact that excessive alcohol intake causes sedation and less physical activity, which again has a negative effect on one's bones, may compound this effect. And there is the additional factor that alcoholics tend not to have a good, balanced diet with a high enough calcium intake. (The problem can be compounded by the fact that alcoholics are prone to falling over when drunk, which creates the opportunity for fractures to occur.)

Steroids

Drugs known as corticosteroids, or just 'steroids' (prednisolone, dexamethasone), result in rapid bone loss – up to a third of the bone mass, within the first three to six months of use. Steroids exert their action mainly on the osteoblasts, so reducing bone formation, and bone resorption by the osteoclasts is also increased. Bone loss is reversible once steroids are withdrawn, although bone strength may not return completely to the level before steroids were started. If steroids are to be used for three months or more, therefore, some osteoporosis protection should be prescribed at the same time. These guidelines on the steroid effect of osteoporosis were agreed only in December 2002 by the Royal College of Physicians (*Glucocorticoid-induced osteoporosis: Guidelines for prevention and treatment*) and so in the past people have been treated with steroids and not given osteoporosis protection.

Steroids are a vital part of medical treatment for a number of conditions, including severe asthma, rheumatological and haematological (blood) conditions, some chemotherapy treatments for cancer, and severe allergies.

Diseases

There are various rare diseases that are also risk factors for osteoporosis. Hormone (endocrine) disorders such as Cushing's syndrome, an overactive thyroid or an over-treated underactive thyroid, or underactive sexual hormones for any reason are associated with low bone mass. Approximately 50 per cent of men with osteoporosis are found to be low in testosterone. Any disease that affects absorption from the gut – for example, coeliac disease (wheat intolerance), chronic liver disease or chronic pancreatitis – can also lower bone density. The inflammatory bowel diseases, ulcerative colitis and Crohn's disease, also increase the risk of osteoporosis. Diseases that are treated with high-dose steroids are mentioned above. Renal and liver failure also cause osteoporosis. Epilepsy and antiepileptic drugs are also risk factors for the development of osteoporosis.

Diagnosis of osteoporosis

Osteoporosis does not show any symptoms until a fracture occurs. However, people at high risk may be assessed by measuring their bone mass. An ordinary X-ray can sometimes suggest thin-looking bones, but it is a very unreliable method of assessing bone density. At present, the 'gold standard' for assessing bone mass at the spine and the hip is the dual energy X-ray absorptiometry (DEXA) scan. Its measurement is a predictive factor for fracture risk. DEXA machines are large and available only in hospitals, although there is a portable mini-DEXA, known as a PIXI, which can be used in the community, and which is undergoing assessment for reliability in large trials. At present the PIXI is thought to be useful at the extremes of bone density: in other words, it predicts well and agrees with a DEXA if bone density is normal or very thin, but it is not as reliable as DEXA in the middle range, where bones are slightly weak and may or may not require treatment. Another alternative is the small portable heel ultrasound, which uses sound waves rather than X-ray radiation. Again, this method is more accurate at the extremes of bone density, and is less reliable in the middle range.

It may be argued that both these small, portable machines are very useful in the community for screening high-risk people because they will give information accurately about approximately two-thirds of the high-risk people screened, which would reduce the number of DEXA scans required. Across 40 per cent of the UK, DEXA scans are not available on request by general practitioners and people have to be referred to a specialist clinic before they can have their bone density measured. This is the greatest stumbling block at present to effective screening for people at high risk of osteoporosis.

Measuring bone density

The World Health Organisation (WHO) has proposed two thresholds for bone mineral density in women, based on the 'T score'. The T score is the value expressed in standard deviation (SD) units from the population mean in young adults. It describes how far the measured bone density is from the average young adult bone density. In this way it measures the relative risk of osteoporosis.

Osteopenia (thin bones) is defined as a T score between –1 and –2.5 and has been proven to be associated with double the increase in fracture risk. Osteoporosis is defined as a T score of less than –2.5 and is linked to four times the risk of fracture, compared with a woman with a normal bone mineral density.

Definition of osteoporosis (WHO criteria)

Bone mineral density – Diagnosis	T score (SD units)	Fracture risk
Normal	less than 1 SD unit below average density for a young adult	low
Osteopenia	1–2.5 units below	above average
Osteoporosis	more than 2.5 SD units below	high
Severe osteoporosis	more than 2.5 SD units below and one or more fractures	already present

Who should have a bone density measurement?

The only point in measuring bone density is that women who are found to have low bone density can be persuaded to accept treatment for it. For this reason, mass-population screening of all menopausal women (similar to mammography to screen for breast cancer), is not considered to be cost effective. The high-risk group – those with three risk factors or a previous fragility (or 'low-impact') fracture – should be targeted. The National Osteoporosis Society (NOS)* has a very effective questionnaire, which can help you assess your own risk with the help of a nurse.

In addition to the detection of osteoporosis by screening, a DEXA scan can also be used for subsequent monitoring of those with osteoporosis. It has been argued that once treatment is started a DEXA scan should be repeated every two to three years to prove that treatment is effective. However, there is a great deal of controversy about this. In some areas of the country DEXA scans are a very limited resource and physicians feel that it is better to screen high-risk people who are not being treated than those already on treatment, who should be improving anyway. On the other hand, it is difficult for patients to take long-term treatment without any evidence that they are getting better. It is also becoming recognised that a small number of people do not respond to a particular treatment, and they need to be identified. It is thought that in the future (see Chapter 11) biochemical 'bone turnover markers' will be used to assess how people respond to treatment, rather than repeating DEXAs.

All men who have suffered a fragility fracture should be referred to specialist clinics for screening.

Treatments for osteoporosis

As is often stated, prevention is better than cure. As mentioned earlier in this chapter, it is of great concern that children of the 21st century have a much lower bone density, owing to their sedentary lifestyle, smoking in their early teens, fizzy-drink consumption and low milk consumption than those of previous generations. It is very important that children are educated about the benefits of a well-balanced diet, rich in calcium; regular weight-bearing exercise, not smoking, and drinking alcohol only in moderation. To ensure that their bone mineral density is maximised in their early twenties and remains so until their forties, teenage girls should not indulge in dieting to extremes.

Summary of drugs used in the treatment of osteoporosis

- Hormone replacement therapy (see Chapter 5)
- Bisphosphonates
- Calcium and vitamin D
- Calcitonin
- Calcitriol
- Parathyroid hormone (PTH)
- Selective oestrogen receptor modulators (SERMs, see Chapter 10)

Hormone replacement therapy

The pros and cons of hormone replacement therapy (HRT) are discussed in Chapter 5. HRT is very effective at preventing bone loss when taken in the perimenopause and postmenopause, as opposed to prior to the menopause. What must be remembered, however, is that HRT is effective for preventing osteoporosis only for as long as it is taken; as soon as the treatment is stopped, the decrease in bone mineral density starts as it would have done from the beginning of the menopause. Therefore if, for example, a woman takes HRT for five years around the age of 50 to improve her menopausal symptoms, the treatment will not have any remaining effect on her bones by the time she gets to 80 and fractures her hip. For this reason the Committee on Safety of

Medicines* has decreed, in December 2003, that HRT should no longer be considered as a first-line treatment for primary osteoporosis prevention. This is because very long-term use of HRT carries an increased risk of breast cancer.

Bisphosphonates

Bisphosphonates are powerful inhibitors of bone resorption. However, one problem is that they are poorly absorbed from the gut and so must be taken on an empty stomach, because the presence of food can reduce their absorption. There are three bisphosphonates currently available: etidronate (Didronel), risedronate (Actonel) and alendronate (Fosamax). All reduce the risk of fractures at the lumbar spine (the lower back). However, only alendronate and risedronate have been shown to reduce the risk of hip fracture. The effect of treatment with these drugs tends to plateau after two years, and at the time of writing it is unclear how long the optimum treatment duration should be, although this is thought to be about five years. These drugs have a very long half-life (the time it takes for half the amount to be excreted from the body) and it is possible that small amounts may remain in the skeleton permanently. It is also unknown what the likely long-term side-effects of these drugs may be, as they have been in use for only about 15 years. As they are not hormonal drugs they can be used equally effectively in men and women with osteoporosis. Preparations are available that need to be taken only once a week, and preparations that would require infusion (slow intravenous) injections once-yearly are being investigated in clinical trials (see Chapter 11).

Calcium and vitamin D

Calcium supplements are often given in addition to other therapies. Calcium alone reduces the rate of bone loss but does not prevent it. In elderly people who are vitamin D deficient because they never go out in sunlight, a supplement of 800 iu (international units) of vitamin D plus 1,000–1,500mg of elemental calcium has been shown to significantly reduce the risk of non-vertebral fracture. Different preparations of calcium and vitamin D can be problematic for different people: for example, the taste and amount of grittiness can vary (the 'grit' can get under the dentures of elderly people), and some fizzy calcium and vitamin D supplements can cause indigestion or diarrhoea for some people. However, there are a number of different preparations available and most individuals can eventually find one that suits his or her taste. These supplements can be bought over the counter, which is often cheaper than a prescription charge.

A quick reference to calcium-rich foods

Weight/volume		Food	Quantity of calcium (mg)
1/3pt	190ml	Skimmed milk	235
1/3pt	190ml	Semi-skimmed milk	231
1/3pt	190ml	Silver-top milk	224
1/3pt	190ml	Soya milk	25
5oz	140g	Low-fat fruit yoghurt	225
1oz	28g	Cheddar cheese	202
1oz	28g	Cottage cheese	82
1oz	28g	Processed cheese	168
3oz	84g	Cheese omelette (1 egg, 1oz Cheddar)	235
3oz	84g	Cheese and egg flan	219
4oz	112g	Cheese and tomato pizza	235
2oz	56g	Sardines, canned in tomato sauce	258
2oz	56g	Pilchards, canned in tomato sauce	168
2oz	56g	Milk chocolate	123
2oz	56g	Mars bar	90
4oz	114g	Spinach, boiled	179
4oz	112g	Broccoli, boiled	45
4oz	112g	Baked beans	59
4oz	112g	Red kidney beans, cooked	80
3oz	84g	Soya bean curd, steamed	428
2oz	56g	Brazil nuts	95
2oz	56g	Swiss style muesli	76
1oz	28g	Dried figs	76
1 slice	30g	Bread, white	33

Source: The National Osteoporosis Society

Calcitonin

Three hormones regulate calcium in the body: calcitonin, calcitriol and parathyroid hormone (PTH). Calcitonin has to be injected under the skin, as if it is taken orally it is digested – broken down – in the gut, rather than being absorbed. A nasal spray is available in the US, but not yet in the UK. Calcitonin is a potent inhibitor of bone resorption and so increases bone mass by 5 per cent over two years, although its ability to reduce fracture remains unclear. It can also be effective in controlling pain associated with osteoporotic vertebral fractures. However, it is an extremely expensive treatment and has severe side-effects of nausea and hot flushes, which patients find extremely unpleasant.

Parathyroid hormone (PTH)

Intermittent PTH therapy (usually by injection) increases bone density and strength. Recent studies have shown that post-menopausal women with osteoporosis who were treated with PTH had a reduced risk of vertebral fractures, although no effect on hip fractures was demonstrated. Further studies are being performed but, again, it is an extremely expensive treatment.

Calcitriol

As with calcitonin and parathyroid hormone, calcitriol is not a standard treatment owing to its expense. Clinical trials are being carried out in the UK.

Selective oestrogen receptor modulators (SERMs)

SERMs are discussed in detail in Chapter 10. It must be remembered that people on tamoxifen, used as a treatment for breast cancer, have an extremely good bone density. Therefore women who are being treated with tamoxifen need not worry about osteoporosis while they are on this medication.

Hip protectors

Hip protectors are large pads – rather like cricket pads but hip shaped – made into knickers. The idea is that they help cushion the hips and reduce fractures when falls are frequent, for example in high-risk elderly women. They have been shown to be effective in clinical trials, but acceptance of them is poor. They are more difficult to get on and off than ordinary knickers, which can be a problem for women with weak or rheumatic hands or those with weak bladder control.

Chapter 4

Heart disease

Heart disease is the biggest cause of death in women in the UK. This chapter outlines the main causes of heart disease and the effect the menopause has on this vital organ.

The structure of the heart

The heart is a large muscle which pumps blood around the body. Veins carry blood from the body to the heart. Small veins join up, and blood enters the heart via two large veins, the superior and inferior vena cava, which bring blood into the right upper chamber of the heart (the right atrium). This blood does not contain much oxygen as the oxygen has been taken up by the cells of the body. The blood passes from the right atrium, down past the tricuspid valve and into the lower right chamber, the right ventricle. The blood leaves the heart by passing through the pulmonary valve and enters the lungs in the pulmonary arteries to collect more oxygen. The purpose of the valves is to keep blood flowing in the proper direction. From the lungs, the blood re-enters the left side of the heart in the pulmonary veins. It flows first into the upper left chamber, the left atrium, past the mitral valve and into the lower left chamber, the left ventricle. From the left ventricle, the blood passes through the aortic valve and is pumped out to the rest of the body and brain. The blood leaving the heart is full of oxygen which it will deliver to the cells of the body. The heart itself has a network of blood vessels which surround it and keep it working well. These are called the coronary arteries.

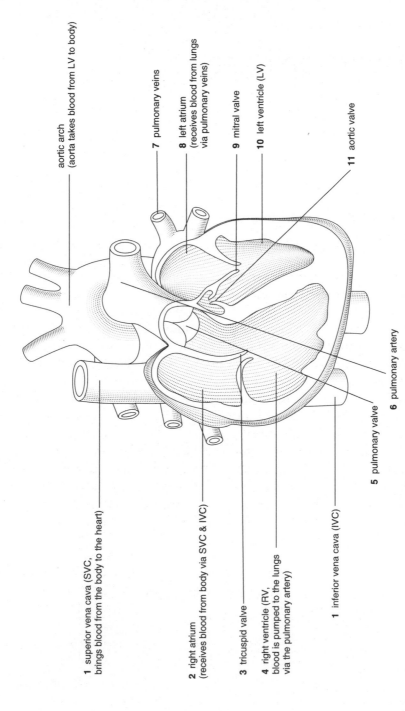

Figure 1 Structure of the heart: 1–11 shows passage of blood through the heart and lungs

aortic arch
(aorta takes blood from LV to body)

7 pulmonary veins

8 left atrium
(receives blood from lungs
via pulmonary veins)

9 mitral valve

10 left ventricle (LV)

11 aortic valve

6 pulmonary artery

5 pulmonary valve

1 inferior vena cava (IVC)

4 right ventricle (RV,
blood is pumped to the lungs
via the pulmonary artery)

3 tricuspid valve

2 right atrium
(receives blood from body via SVC & IVC)

1 superior vena cava (SVC,
brings blood from the body to the heart)

Causes of heart disease

Ischaemic heart disease

Ischaemic heart disease results from the narrowing of the coronary arteries such that the blood supply to the heart is impaired. In this condition, the heart muscle does not get enough blood when it is working hard, so the person experiences a chest pain when undergoing physical exertion. This is similar to muscle cramp in any other overworked muscle, but if the heart gets cramp it is known as **angina**. If a heart vessel becomes completely blocked then the section of heart muscle supplied by that vessel dies: this is called a heart attack or myocardial infarction. A heart attack causes chest pain at rest, although occasionally it may be completely symptomless (or 'silent'). People who are diabetic are more likely to have silent heart attacks.

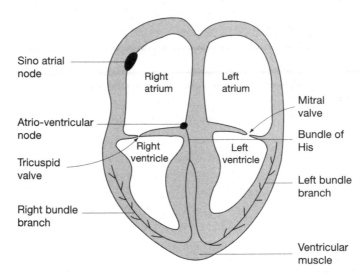

Figure 2 The chambers of the heart with the electrical conduction system

Problems of rhythm

The heart has an electrical wiring system made up of nerves that send out pulses of electrical discharge through the muscle of the heart so that the muscular contraction is smoothly coordinated to maximise the efficiency of each heartbeat. The bundle of nerves in the atria where the initial electrical impulse takes place is called the pacemaker. The nerves that then take the electrical impulse round the rest of the heart to organise the contraction for each beat are known as the electrical bundles. People can be born with problems in the electrical wiring of the heart or it can occur with age. Many people experience extra heartbeats, known as atrial extrasytolic beats, which are completely safe but very disconcerting.

During the menopause it is very common to get palpitations or an irregular heartbeat because of the hormonal chaos that is occurring. Women may be concerned about these palpitations and sometimes feel that they are about to die. Fortunately, these palpitations are usually completely harmless.

Doctors sometimes recommend a simple 24-hour recording of the heart to check on what is causing the palpitations. Electrodes are put on the chest and a recording is made of the heart throughout a 24-hour period during which the person goes about her normal activities. She is asked to press a button every time she experiences certain symptoms so that the cardiologist can correlate the symptoms to any possible changes in rhythm recorded by the monitor. This is extremely helpful as often people experience symptoms without a change in rhythm, and sometimes people have a serious change in rhythm without any symptoms. Occasionally the two correlate. The 24-hour tape can usually sift those people with completely harmless extra beats (up to 33 per cent of the population experience these from time to time) from the tiny minority of people who do have a serious electrical conduction problem, known as heart block. Those who are found to have a problem can be offered a variety of different treatments (medical, surgical and electrical) depending on the exact nature of the electrical fault.

Valvular disease

There are four important valves in the heart which stop the blood flowing backwards when the heart muscle contracts. If the valves are not closing completely a small amount of blood squirts backwards at each contraction, which reduces the efficiency of the heart. Occasionally, valves can leak so badly or be so tight that they do not open or shut properly, which puts the person at risk. People who

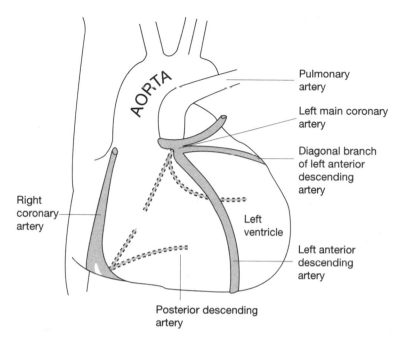

Figure 3 The coronary arteries

have this condition experience extreme breathlessness when carrying out trivial tasks such as talking or getting dressed. A valve replacement may be considered for them.

At the start of the twentieth century in the UK, when rheumatic disease was common in children, a frequent long-term side-effect was damage to the valves of the heart. This has fortunately become very rare in the UK in anyone born after the 1930s. A much more common problem now is mitral valve prolapse. One in ten people has a slightly floppy mitral valve which wiggles during the heartbeat. This can cause turbulence which is transmitted as a noise called a heart murmur. Occasionally doctors pick up these heart murmurs when listening with a stethoscope. People with a floppy mitral valve need antibiotics when having surgical procedures such as dentistry or in childbirth, because they are slightly more likely to get bacteria growing on the floppy valve, leading to an infection called subacute bacterial endocarditis (SBE). They otherwise can lead a completely normal life.

Atrial fibrillation

The normal heartbeat is regular and occurs between 60 and 80 times per minute in an adult. This is known as sinus rhythm. For various reasons some people develop an irregular heartbeat – one type is known as atrial fibrillation. People with this condition can feel slightly more breathless even when at rest because their heart is not beating efficiently. Atrial fibrillation is more common in people who have an overactive thyroid (thyrotoxicosis).

People with atrial fibrillation are slightly more likely to suffer a stroke because clots can form in the chambers of the heart owing to turbulence patterns. The clot can then travel from the heart up into the brain arteries causing a vascular blockage, or stroke. People with atrial fibrillation are therefore often advised to take warfarin, a medication that thins down the blood and which has been shown to lower the risks of strokes. Other drugs, such as digoxin or sotalol, can slow down the rhythm, so allowing the heart to beat more efficiently. A person whose atrial fibrillation is recent may be given a huge electrical shock to the heart to convert its rhythm back to the normal sinus rhythm again. This is known as electrical cardioversion, and for obvious reasons has to be performed in hospital with trained cardiologists present.

Cholesterol

Cholesterol is a major risk factor for coronary heart disease. It is a fat in the blood which produces hormones; excess levels of it may cause deposits which can block blood vessels and cause heart disease. It is estimated that half the population of the UK have a cholesterol level that puts them at significant risk of heart disease. However, cholesterol must not be thought of in isolation, as a number of other major risk factors contribute to heart disease including smoking, diabetes mellitus, family history and a raised blood pressure. Unfortunately, all these risk factors multiply together to increase the risk. If someone has already had a heart attack or is diabetic, the aim is to get the cholesterol level below 5mmol per litre (the average blood cholesterol for women in the UK is 5.9mmol per litre; this rises with age so that by the age of 55, three out of four women have cholesterol levels over 6.5mmol per litre).

As mentioned above, cholesterol is an essential fatty molecule that is used in the body to make steroid hormones. The fats are actually divided into two different molecules: low density lipoproteins (LDL) and high density lipoproteins (HDL). High levels of LDL are predictors of coronary heart disease, whereas high levels of HDL appear to be protective. Triglycerides, another component of cholesterol, are also important, and if they are high people are at risk of pancreatitis.

Indicators of high cholesterol levels

Xanthoma are yellow deposits of fat in the skin usually around the eyes, just under the eyebrows, which can indicate a high level of cholesterol in the body. Sometimes people have a whitish deposit in the iris of their eye which can be seen as a pale arc in the iris (corneal arcus), which can also be a sign of high levels of cholesterol. For most people a high level of cholesterol in the body is completely without symptoms. The only way of knowing the level is by taking a fasting blood test. Fasting means that the person does not eat anything from 10pm the previous night if blood is taken at 8.30am the next morning. Diabetics need to discuss the procedure beforehand to make sure their blood sugar levels do not fall too low by being kept waiting at the surgery. Acceptable levels of cholesterol have been radically revised downwards over the last ten years. If a person has had a heart attack or is diabetic it is recommended that the cholesterol level be below 5mmol per litre.

How to reduce the risks of heart disease

Everyone can take steps to lower their cholesterol levels. The following are the most important factors in lowering the risks of ischaemic heart disease:

- maintaining a low body weight (lose weight if obese)
- eating a low-fat Mediterranean diet
- avoiding alcohol
- stopping smoking
- treating diabetes mellitus
- treating blood pressure adequately
- taking at least 30 minutes of exercise three to four times a week.

The importance of stopping smoking cannot be overemphasised. It is the most important risk factor in heart disease, and many GPs run support clinics for those wanting to give up the habit, with trained counsellors and medication such as nicotine patches or tablets that help people to stop smoking.

Statins

A group of drugs known as statins have changed the rate of heart disease over the last decade by dramatically reducing cholesterol levels. The only major (but rare) side-effect is that some people get muscular aches and pains. Muscle enzymes should be monitored in the first six weeks of starting a statin, and the drug should be stopped if the enzyme levels become abnormal. Statins have now been granted an 'over the counter' licence in the UK, so that they are not prescription-only, but available to buy at pharmacies, although how this will be regulated remains unclear at present. Examples of statins are simvastatin (Zocor), atorvastatin (Lipitor), fluvastatin (Lescol) and pravastatin (Lipostat).

Blood pressure

Blood pressure is a measurement of the pressure in the arteries when the surge of blood is at its greatest (systolic), and when the heart is relaxing to fill up with blood so the pressure drops to its lowest reading (diastolic). That is why there are two readings: for example, 140/60. The view on the management of blood pressure has changed appreciably in the last 20 years, with the level at which treatment should begin dropping lower and lower. This is because rigorous studies have shown that even a small fall in blood pressure reduces the risk of strokes and heart attacks. In high-risk groups, such as diabetics or people who already have had a heart attack or stroke, it is even more important. Ten years ago, GPs were aiming to bring the population's blood pressure below 160/95. Now the national target in the new GP contract is 150/90, and 140/85 in high-risk groups.

Blood pressure tends to rise naturally with age, and so it should be checked every five years. There is a genetic element to high blood pressure. Also, women who have had high blood pressure in pregnancy, known as toxaemia or pre-eclampsia, are much more at risk of developing high blood pressure in middle age, even though the blood pressure had gone back to normal after the baby was born.

Most cases of high blood pressure are completely asymptomatic. Because they experience no signs, people can have high blood pressure for years without realising it. The only way to find out is to get a check-up. If you are seeing your doctor for some other issue and know you have not had your blood pressure checked for a number of years, ask for it to be checked.

There are many different drugs used to lower blood pressure. Some people experience side-effects, but because of the wide range of medicines available, one can usually be found to suit the individual. See *The Which? Guide to Women's Health* for general advice on lowering blood pressure and *Which? Medicine* for details of drugs used to treat the condition.

Clots

A blood clot in the deep veins of the leg or pelvis is called a deep vein thrombosis (DVT). This is different from a clot or inflammation in the superficial or surface veins of the leg, which is often called superficial thrombophlebitis. The danger of a deep vein thrombosis is that the clot can travel up through the veins into the lung causing acute sharp chest pain on breathing in, pleuritic chest pain and breathlessness. Large blood clots in the lung (pulmonary emboli or PEs) are life-threatening.

The physiology of clotting

The clotting mechanism (or cascade) is an immensely complex pathway which allows our blood to circulate around our bodies but also to form a clot at the exposed surface if we cut ourselves so that we do not immediately bleed to death. It therefore has immense survival evolutionary significance. It is believed that at about the last Ice Age a mutation occurred in the clotting cascade which caused people to clot slightly more quickly. This had an evolutionary advantage in that they were less likely to bleed to death in childbirth, or in accidents or fights. This one genetic mutation spread rapidly through the Northern European population, so that now one in 20 people in the UK is affected. This mutation, discovered in Leiden in 1993, is known as Leiden V. People with Leiden V mutation are more likely to clot, and so develop a DVT or PE. However, a lot of people who have DVT have no recognised clotting abnormality. This may simply mean that that particular clotting abnormality has yet to be discovered.

For the increased risks of DVT and PE from taking HRT see Chapter 5.

Risks factors for deep vein thrombosis and pulmonary emboli

Conditions that increase the chances of DVT or PE include:

- abnormal clotting factors
- pregnancy
- childbirth
- surgery to the pelvis
- surgery to the hip or knee
- smoking
- the combined oral contraceptive pill
- HRT (see Chapter 5)
- immobility
- long-haul flight (over six hours)
- strong family history
- previous history of PE or clots
- cancer
- obesity.

Chapter 5

Hormone replacement therapy

If menopausal and postmenopausal symptoms disrupt your life you may wish to take an external supply of hormones to replace the body's dwindling ovarian supplies of oestrogen and progesterone. This is called hormone replacement therapy (HRT), a term that is most usually associated with replacing female hormones, but also applies to the replacement of other body hormones when there are deficiencies, for example with thyroid or adrenal problems. Although the ovaries cease to produce female hormones at the menopause, a tiny amount is still produced by the adrenal glands.

Before starting HRT you should discuss with your doctor the pros and cons of using it and what type of preparation might help. HRT has been widely used to prevent osteoporosis in women over 50 years of age, but is now reserved as second-line treatment. More information on the long-term benefits and risks of using HRT has become available from large-scale studies in the UK and in North America (see box on page 83) that have helped to place HRT in perspective. In summary, the majority of medical experts consider that:

- for short-term treatment of menopausal symptoms the balance of risks and benefits is favourable and HRT therefore remains a suitable treatment option. The lowest effective dose should be used for the shortest possible time, and treatment should be reviewed at least once a year
- for long-term use for preventing osteoporosis the balance of risks and benefits is unfavourable. HRT should be used for preventing osteoporosis only by those who are unable to take other treatments for the condition or for whom other treatments have been unsuccessful

- in women who have experienced a premature menopause, HRT can be used for treating menopausal symptoms and for preventing osteoporosis until the age of 50 years. After 50 years the choice of therapy for preventing osteoporosis should be reviewed by your doctor
- in healthy women without symptoms, the balance of risks and benefits is generally unfavourable and HRT is not recommended.

The benefits and risks of HRT are discussed in more detail later in the chapter. Once you have read them all, you will need to decide for yourself whether or not to start HRT.

Ways of taking HRT

HRT is available as **combined therapy** or as **oestrogen-only**. Combined therapy, which must be taken if you have a womb (uterus), comes in two types – *sequential combined* and *continuous combined HRT*. If you have already had your uterus removed (hysterectomy) you can take oestrogen on its own: you do not need to add progestogen.

Combined therapy

Low doses of an oestrogen are given with a progestogen, a synthetic equivalent of progesterone, for 10–14 days each 28-day cycle to protect the uterus from changes in its lining (endometrium) brought about by the oestrogen. The cyclical use of progestogen leads to withdrawal bleeding, a 'pseudo' period, at the end of a month or three months, although around one woman in 20 does not bleed on a monthly cycle.

When HRT was introduced in the 1950s women were prescribed oestrogen on its own for menopausal symptoms even when they had a uterus. By the 1960s it was clear that oestrogen could cause a thickening of the uterine lining (endometrial hyperplasia) through an increase in the number of endometrial cells. Endometrial hyperplasia itself is not a cancerous condition, but it can lead to the development of endometrial cancer. Progestogen is therefore given for part of each cycle to oppose the effects of oestrogen on the uterus.

Sequential combined HRT

This is a combination of oestrogen usually taken continuously and progestogen taken cyclically during a one-month or three-month cycle. Oestrogen is sometimes used cyclically for 21 out of 28 days: the last week is oestrogen-free, which means that menopausal symptoms can return during this week. Monthly sequential combined HRT is suitable if you have a womb and you still have periods (perimenopausal). Either monthly or three-monthly sequential combined HRT is suitable if your last period was less than a year ago. Regular bleeding can be a nuisance but it is important to take progestogen to protect the endometrium (see 'Progestogen preparations' below).

Continuous combined HRT

When you are definitely postmenopausal, a year or more after the end of your periods, you can take oestrogen and progestogen continuously on a daily basis. If you take continuous combined HRT within a year of your periods stopping you may experience irregular bleeding at the start of treatment. Continued irregular bleeding needs investigation and you should see your doctor for a check-up. If you are taking hormonal preparations already, including the oral contraceptive pill, and want to start continuous combined HRT, it may be difficult to determine whether or not you are postmenopausal because periods have been halted by hormonal treatment. However, eight out of ten women are post-menopausal by the age of 54 years.

Oestrogen-only

Oestrogen-only HRT is suitable if you have had a hysterectomy and your uterus has been removed. If the uterus has been removed totally then no endometrium remains and any external source of oestrogen can be given without the risk of endometrial hyperplasia developing. (Oestrogen stimulates endometrial growth and therefore must be used on its own only when the endometrium has been removed or totally destroyed, otherwise a progestogen must be added as in combined HRT.)

Choice of replacement hormones

Oestrogens

Natural oestrogens (that is, those derived from animals or plants), such as estradiol, estriol and estrone, are generally used in HRT because they are considered to be better than synthetic alternatives (that is, those made entirely in the laboratory), ethinylestradiol or mestranol, which have a greater effect on the body's metabolism. Ethinylestradiol was used previously as HRT for menopausal symptoms. It is widely used in oral contraceptives.

Yams and soya beans are used to derive estradiol, estriol or estrone and so these are partially synthesised. Conjugated oestrogens, derived from the urine of pregnant mares, contain estrone sulphate and other equine oestrogens, mainly equilin. Conjugated oestrogens, for example in Premarin and Prempak-C, are widely used, particularly in North American clinical trials of HRT.

The main unwanted effects of oestrogen include feeling sick, vomiting, retention of fluid in the body, bloating, abdominal cramps, weight change, and tenderness and enlargement of the breasts. Other side-effects include changes in sexual drive (libido), headache, migraine, dizziness, leg cramps, depression, irritation of contact lenses and, rarely, the development of jaundice, skin rashes and patchy brown discolouration of the skin (chloasma).

Progestogens

There are two main groups of progestogen in use for HRT that are similar to and capable of replacing the body's hormone, progesterone. Dydrogesterone and medroxyprogesterone are based on progesterone, while norethisterone, norgestrel and its relative levonorgestrel are derived from testosterone, the male hormone. Both male and female sex hormones are derived from one body chemical, cholesterol, and the variation of effect comes from the way different chemical groupings are attached to the cholesterol molecule when these hormones are made in the body.

If HRT containing one type of progestogen does not suit you, then changing to a preparation with a different progestogen may sort out unwanted effects. Progestogens derived from testosterone can sometimes produce androgenic effects, for example acne and excess hair growth (hirsutism). Menopausal women are some-times treated with testosterone, by implant, with HRT. Your hormone profile is unique to you and any one HRT preparation can produce variations in the overall effect, including unwanted effects that you experience. Unwanted effects of progestogen include premenstrual-like tension (retention of fluid in the body, bloating, breast tenderness), menstrual disturbances, weight gain, nausea, vomiting, headache, dizziness, difficulty getting to sleep, drowsiness, depression, and skin reactions including nettle rash, itching, rash and acne, extra hair growth and baldness. It may be tempting not to take progestogen especially because of premen-strual tension (PMT), but changing the type of HRT, for example from tablets to the patch, can sometimes lessen progestogen's unwanted effects.

Tibolone

Tibolone (Livial) is a unique preparation for postmenopausal women – it is a synthetic hormonal steroid treatment combining the effects of oestrogen, progestogen and testosterone. It should not be started until one year after the last natural period, and it can be used for relieving postmenopausal symptoms caused by oestrogen deficiency such as hot flushes, sweating and decreased interest in sex. If you have a surgical or premature menopause, you can start tibolone straight away. Similarly, if you are being treated with a gonadotrophin-releasing hormone analogue, for example for endometriosis, then you can start tibolone immediately.

If tibolone is taken within a year of your final period, irregular vaginal bleeding may occur. The progestogenic activity of tibolone should protect the endometrium, and you do not have to take any additional progestogen. There should be no monthly bleeding, but occasionally bleeding or spotting may occur, mainly during the first few months of treatment. If you do experience continued vaginal bleeding, discuss this with your doctor. Tibolone is taken once a day as a single 2.5 milligram (mg) tablet on a continuous basis.

Tibolone can also be used to prevent osteoporosis from a year after the menopause if you are at high risk of fractures, but only if you cannot take or tolerate other first-line treatments for osteoporosis.

Unwanted effects occur occasionally and include changes in body weight, dizziness, skin reactions such as itching, rashes and dermatitis, headache, increased hair growth on the face and fluid retention.

The risk of breast cancer increases with the use of tibolone compared with no HRT use, although the risk is lower with tibolone than with combined HRT. Endometrial hyperplasia and endometrial cancer have occasionally been reported in women taking tibolone, although it is not clear whether they are caused by tibolone.

Types of HRT preparations

Combined oestrogen and progestogen preparations

Combined HRT can be taken in a number of different ways, for example with oestrogen and progestogen in the same tablet or patch, or an oestrogen-only preparation (such as a gel) with progestogen tablets for part of each cycle. It is important to find a preparation or several products that you can use easily so that you do not forget to take the progestogen element each month. The advantages and disadvantages of the different types of HRT are summarised in Table F on page 77.

When oestrogen and progestogen are presented in one pack as two different medicines (as for example in sequential combined HRT, see below), you have to pay two prescription charges. Continuous combined preparations are now formulated with oestrogen and progestogen in one tablet or patch, and you have to pay for only one prescription. If you use different types of HRT, for example gel and tablets, then you will pay two prescription charges.

Sequential combined tablets

Preparations of oestrogen are now taken continuously, repeating the 28-day cycles, with a progestogen added for 10–14 days of each cycle and preferably for at least 12 days. Older preparations, such as Cyclo-Progynova, are taken for only 21 days, followed by a seven-day break. Symptoms may return during this week, and for this reason oestrogen is more usually taken for 28 days and continued without interruption. Estradiol is the main oestrogen used in tablets, although conjugated oestrogens are also used in Prempak-C and Premique Cycle. A choice of progestogens is available (see Table A).

Table A: Sequential combined HRT

Brand name	Oestrogen	Progestogen	Number of days progestogen	Type
CLIMAGEST	Estradiol	Norethisterone	12	Tablets
CYCLO-PROGYNOVA	Estradiol	Levonorgestrel	10	Tablets
ELLESTE DUET	Estradiol	Norethisterone	12	Tablets
ESTRACOMBI	Estradiol	Norethisterone	14	Patches
EVOREL-PAK	Estradiol	Norethisterone	12	Oestrogen patches with progestogen tablets
EVOREL-SEQUI	Estradiol	Norethisterone	14	Patches
FEMAPAK	Estradiol	Dydrogesterone	14	Oestrogen patches with progestogen tablets
FEMOSTON	Estradiol	Dydrogesterone	14	Tablets
FEMSEVEN SEQUI	Estradiol	Levonorgestrel	14	Patches
FEMTAB SEQUI	Estradiol	Levonorgestrel	12	Tablets
NOVOFEM	Estradiol	Norethisterone	12	Tablets
NUVELLE	Estradiol	Levonorgestrel	12	Tablets
PREMIQUE CYCLE	Conjugated oestrogens	Medroxy-progesterone	14	Tablets
PREMPAK-C	Conjugated oestrogens	Norgestrel	12	Tablets
TRIDESTRA	Estradiol	Medroxy-progesterone	14	Tablets
TRISEQUENS	Estradiol	Norethisterone	10	Tablets

If you are menopausal and still having periods, you can start on day 1 of your menstrual cycle. Many preparations are started then, but others such as Cyclo-Progynova, FemTab Sequi, Nuvelle and Trisequens are started on day 5. If your periods have stopped or are infrequent, you can start HRT tablets at any time. If you are switching from sequential combined HRT with cyclical progestogen, that is with monthly bleeds, to continuous combined HRT with continuous progestogen, then you start this at the end of the scheduled bleed.

Tridestra is the only HRT to combine estradiol valerate (2mg) with medroxyprogesterone (20mg) to produce bleeding every 13 weeks instead of the usual monthly withdrawal bleeding. Estradiol is taken daily for ten weeks (white tablets) followed by two weeks of estradiol plus medroxyprogesterone 20mg (blue tablets) daily, and then one week without hormone treatment when bleeding occurs. Yellow tablets, which are inactive (placebo), are taken during this week to maintain the tablet-taking habit. Premenstrual symptoms are reduced to four times a year as are unwanted and annoying withdrawal bleeds.

Combined patches

A number of preparations (Estracombi, Evorel Sequi, FemSeven Sequi) are complete patch systems providing oestrogen plus two weeks of progestogen per month. (For details of the skin patch formulation see below.)

Tablets and patches

Some preparations (such as Evorel-Pak and Femapak) are available as estradiol patches with progestogen tablets (see Table A).

Combined HRT does not provide effective contraception, nor should it be taken at the same time as an oral contraceptive. Another non-hormonal method of contraception should be chosen if it is needed (see Chapter 7). Fertility can continue after your final menstrual period for two years if you are aged under 50 years and for one year if you are aged over 50 years. If you are aged under 50 years and oral contraception is considered suitable (that is, you have no risk factors for developing blood clots in the veins or arteries), then the combined oral contraceptive pill with a low-dose oestrogen, such as Loestrin 20 or Mercilon, may be suitable. This strategy will provide effective contraception and also relief from menopausal symptoms. Generally, oral contraception can be used to the age of 50, but then other methods should be considered.

Continuous combined preparations

These are mainly tablet formulations, but two patch presentations are available, Evorel-Conti and FemSeven Conti (see Table B). Continuous combined preparations can be started only once you are sure that you are at least one year beyond your final period. Spotting or irregular bleeding can occur especially at the start of treatment. If this continues you must see your doctor as endometrial changes are a possibility and you will need a check-up.

Table B: Continuous combined oestrogen and progestogen (unsuitable for use within 12 months of final menstrual period)

Brand name	Oestrogen	Progestogen	Type
CLIMESSE	Estradiol	Norethisterone	Tablets
ELLESTE-DUET CONTI	Estradiol	Norethisterone	Tablets
EVOREL-CONTI	Estradiol	Norethisterone	Patches
FEMOSTON CONTI	Estradiol	Dydrogesterone	Tablets
FEMSEVEN CONTI	Estradiol	Levonorgestrel	Patches
FEMTAB CONTINUOUS	Estradiol	Norethisterone	Tablets
INDIVINA	Estradiol	Medroxyprogesterone	Tablets
KLIOFEM	Estradiol	Norethisterone	Tablets
KLIOVANCE	Estradiol	Norethisterone	Tablets
NUVELLE CONTINUOUS	Estradiol	Norethisterone	Tablets
PREMIQUE	Conjugated oestrogens	Medroxyprogesterone Tablets	
PREMIQUE LOW DOSE	Conjugated oestrogens	Medroxyprogesterone	Tablets

Oestrogen-only preparations

There is a good choice of oestrogen preparations, mainly of those containing estradiol, the principal oestrogen produced in the ovaries. Most commonly oestrogen is taken by mouth in tablet form, but it can also be applied via the skin in a patch or gel, given as an implant, used in the nose or locally in the vagina as a cream, pessaries or in a ring device. As mentioned earlier in the chapter, an oestrogen–only preparation is suitable on its own only if you have had a hysterectomy. Otherwise, you must take a progestogen for 10–14 days of each 28-day cycle to counteract the effects of oestrogen on the endometrium.

Tablets

Tablets are convenient and are usually packed in a 28-day pack, sometimes with the days of the week marked to remind you to take the daily dose. Three months' supply is often prescribed to allow time for you to become established on the product. Estradiol valerate is commonly used in a range of tablet preparations, but conjugated oestrogens, estrone and estriol are also used (see Table C). Estropipate (piperazine estrone sulphate) is a semi-synthetic oestrogen; estrone is responsible for its action.

When taken by mouth, estradiol is released from the tablet and absorbed from the gut into the bloodstream, which transports it to the liver. In the liver, estradiol is converted to the less potent oestrogens, estrone and estriol. Higher doses of oestrogen are needed when you take HRT by mouth to achieve a satisfactory blood level of estradiol. The passage through the liver to convert estradiol to the other oestrogens, known as the first pass effect, can result in unwanted effects being more troublesome.

Several strengths of estradiol are available, mainly as 1mg or 2mg tablets; the lowest dose that relieves your symptoms should always be used. Low doses of estradiol are not effective in preventing osteoporosis: for example, Zumenon tablets containing 1mg of estradiol are used for menopausal symptoms only, whereas Zumenon containing 2mg of estradiol can be used for menopausal symptoms and to prevent osteoporosis where HRT use is appropriate for osteoporosis prevention (say, if you have a premature menopause). An asterisk is used in Table C to indicate those tablet preparations and strengths that can be used to prevent osteoporosis for which they must be taken continuously.

Table C: Oestrogen-only tablets

Brand name	Daily dose	Oestrogen
CLIMAVAL	1–2mg	Estradiol valerate
ELLESTE SOLO	1–2*mg	Estradiol
FEMTAB	1–2*mg	Estradiol valerate
HARMOGEN*	1.5–3mg	Estropipate
HORMONIN*	1–2 tablets	Estradiol + estriol + estrone
OVESTIN	0.5–3mg for up to 1 month, then 0.5–1mg	Estriol
PREMARIN*	0.625–1.25mg	Conjugated oestrogens
PROGYNOVA	1–2*mg	Estradiol valerate
ZUMENON	1–2*mg	Estradiol valerate

* For menopausal symptoms and to prevent osteoporosis.

Skin patches

A skin patch is another way of delivering hormones to your body. Estradiol is incorporated in adhesive base on one side of a patch or plaster which, when applied to the skin, releases the drug gradually and through the skin (transdermally) into the bloodstream. The transdermal route avoids estradiol passing through the liver, so lower doses of the hormone can control symptoms than would be the case with tablets. Moreover, unwanted effects such as nausea may be less troublesome.

Doses of estradiol range from 25 to 100 micrograms (mcg), and a starting dose of 40 or 50mcg is recommended for the first month of therapy which can be adjusted to the lowest effective dose that controls symptoms in subsequent months. Each dose is released from the patch into the body over a 24-hour period (see Table D). The dose of estradiol needs to be adequate to prevent osteoporosis, and low doses of oestrogen (for example, Elleste Solo MX 40mcg or Estraderm MX or TTS 25mcg) do not provide this protection. Progestogen must be added if you have not had a hysterectomy, and it can be taken as tablets or in a patch (see 'Combined oestrogen and progestogen preparations').

Using the patch

For some preparations (FemSeven and Progynova TS preparations) the patch is used once a week, and for others (see Table D) twice a week either continuously or on a cyclical basis depending on your requirements. The twice-weekly patches must be changed every three to four days and it is easier to remember to do this on the same two days each week. For example, if you start your HRT course on a Monday you should change the patch on Thursday that week and then again on Monday of the following week and then Thursday. Your patch-changing days are then fixed for Monday and Thursday every week. If you forget to change the patch or it comes off, then apply another patch as soon as possible and continue with your original patch-changing routine. If you use an oestrogen patch on a cyclical basis then you have a patch-free interval for one week in four. Menopausal symptoms may return during this week, so most oestrogen skin patch products are used continuously.

The patch must be placed on a clean, dry hairless area of unbroken skin free of cuts, spots and other skin blemishes, and not on skin which you have just moisturised with cream or applied talc to. Instructions will be provided with the patch in the form of the manufacturer's patient information leaflet which should tell you how to remove the patch from its wrapping and how to apply it. The patch should be placed on skin below the waist, for example on your bottom or thigh. It should never be placed on or near the breasts. Avoid placing the patch under elasticated waistbands or where clothes rub the body.

Skin reactions such as redness, itching and rash can occur but they generally fade when the patch is removed, so a different site should be used each time it is changed. If skin reactions persist then you should remove the patch and discuss the problems with your doctor. The adhesive used in skin patches now causes fewer allergic skin reactions than the earlier patch products, but nevertheless reactions can still occur. Unwanted hormonal effects that may occur include headaches, breast tenderness, stomach pain and bloating and irregular vaginal bleeding, particularly at the start of HRT.

The patch can be kept on when bathing or showering, but avoid loosening its edges. When changing the patch avoid applying the patch immediately after a hot bath or shower: wait for the skin to cool down. You can also swim with the patch on and exercise, although you should ensure that clothing does not rub the patch area. When sunbathing, keep the patch covered out of direct sunlight. If the patch leaves a residue of adhesive on the skin after you have removed it, you can use baby oil to help to take these marks off. Get rid of your old patches safely. When you change the patch, take the old one off, fold the sticky side of the patch together and place it in the empty patch wrapper from the new patch. Collect these and then take them to your local pharmacy for disposal, for example when you need your next HRT prescription. Old patches still contain some active oestrogen and should be kept away from children, men and the environment.

Table D: Oestrogen-only patch and gel preparations

Oestrogen-only patches: brand name	Approximate dose of estradiol in micrograms (mcg)/ 24 hours	Patch change routine
ELLESTE-SOLO MX	40, 80*	Twice weekly
ESTRADERM MX	25, 50*, 75*,100	Twice weekly
ESTRADERM TTS	25, 50*, 100	Twice weekly
EVOREL	25, 50*, 75*,100*	Twice weekly
FEMATRIX	40, 80*	Twice weekly
FEMSEVEN	50*, 75*,100*	Once a week
PROGYNOVA TS	50*, 100*	Once a week
Oestrogen-only gels: brand name	Dose	Gel use
OESTROGEL*	1.5mg/two measures (2.5g)	Once a day
SANDRENA	500mcg–1mg	Once a day

For menopausal symptoms and osteoporosis prevention

Skin gels

Skin gels (such as Oestrogel and Sandrena) are an alternative way of giving estradiol transdermally to produce an effect in the body. The gels are applied once daily on a continuous basis; progestogen must be taken for 10–12 days each cycle if you have not had a hysterectomy.

Oestrogel

Oestrogel is an estradiol gel in a pump pack providing 64 doses of 1.25g measures of gel. Each measure contains 750mcg of estradiol. The usual starting dose is two measures (2.5g) of Oestrogel applied once a day, which is equivalent to 1.5mg estradiol (i.e. 2 × 750mcg.)

The lowest effective dose should be used, and if after one month effective relief of menopausal symptoms has not been achieved the dose can be increased up to four measures daily (5g), equivalent to 3mg estradiol. Oestrogel can also be used to prevent osteoporosis.

The gel must be applied to clean dry unbroken skin, for example on the arms and shoulders, or inner thighs, to cover an area at least twice that of the template provided with the pack. One measure, or half the prescribed dose if more than two measures are used, should be applied to one arm or inner thigh and allowed to dry for five minutes before the skin is covered with clothing. The application is repeated for the remainder of the dose.

It may be tempting to seek help with the gel application, but only you should apply it, and skin contact with another person – particularly with a male partner – should be avoided for one hour after application. Oestrogel must not be applied on or near breasts or on the vulval area. Washing the skin or contact with other skin products should be avoided for at least one hour after applying the gel. Using other skin products at the same place as Oestrogel could affect the absorption of estradiol across the skin and reduce its effectiveness. Such products include skin cleansers and detergents, skin preparations containing alcohol (for example, astringents and sunscreens), and products containing salicyclic or lactic acid. Other medicines that alter the natural cycle of skin production, for example some cancer treatments, will affect Oestrogel therapy.

Skin reactions such as irritation and reddening of the skin where you apply the gel can occur occasionally. Using a different site of application helps to overcome this, but if skin reactions continue then discuss them with your doctor. Other unwanted effects of estradiol could include breast tenderness and headache.

Sandrena gel

Sandrena gel is packed in single-dose sachets containing either 500mcg or 1mg estradiol in an alcoholic gel base. The usual starting dose is 1mg estradiol equivalent to 1g gel, but the dose depends on the severity of the symptoms. The dose can be adjusted after 2–3 cycles but usually lies within the range of 500mcg to 1.5mg estradiol per day (0.5g to 1.5g gel per day or one to three sachets). Sandrena can be used for menopausal symptoms, but not for preventing osteoporosis.

Sandrena is applied once daily on intact skin to areas below the waist, such as the thighs, using the right side on one day and then the left side the day afterwards and continuing to alternate sides. The gel should be applied over an area roughly twice the size of a hand. It should not be applied on the breasts, on the face or irritated skin. After application you should allow the gel to dry for a few minutes and avoid washing the application site within one hour. Wash hands after application and take care not to get the gel in the eyes as it may irritate them. Skin irritation can occur where you apply the gel; it contains propylene glycol and ethanol, which can cause allergies. The commonest unwanted effect with Sandrena is breast tenderness.

If you miss a dose, apply the gel as soon as you remember if it is within 12 hours of the missed dose. If the dose is more than 12 hours late, skip the missed dose and continue with the next dose as normal. Breakthrough bleeding may occur if you miss doses. A small plastic box is provided which holds a seven-day supply of sachets to help you to remember to use the daily dose. Some women prefer to use HRT gel daily, but it is more messy and the daily dose must be maintained. Others prefer the patch, once or twice weekly, but women need to get used to the patch-changing routine. If you need to take progestogen for part of the month you will also need to have a system to remind you to take it.

Implants

Implants are long-acting oestrogen preparations containing estradiol which are inserted under the skin (subcutaneously). The implant, about the size of a small pea, is inserted in the fatty tissue below the skin surface of the abdominal wall or the thigh in a simple procedure under local anaesthetic. Once in place the implant releases the hormone continuously into the body over a period of months. Using an implant is similar to the transdermal route in that the replacement hormone bypasses the liver and unwanted effects are less troublesome. Estradiol implants are available in 25, 50 or 100mg strengths and can be used to replace oestrogen and to prevent osteoporosis. The usual starting dose is 25mg or 50mg.

An implant provides the body with estradiol for four to eight months and must then be replaced, depending on when menopausal symptoms return as the oestrogen blood level falls. Major swings in the estradiol blood level can occur with implant usage and yearly measurement of estradiol blood levels is recommended. If the estradiol blood level is gradually increasing, the interval between implant renewal should be increased or the dose reduced. Menopausal symptoms may reappear even when estradiol blood levels should be sufficient for symptom control. This can lead to the use of ever higher doses of estradiol, a phenomenon called 'tachyphylaxis'. The body appears to develop tolerance to estradiol and the effect of the drug gradually diminishes so that escalating doses are needed to control menopausal symptoms. If this happens the dose must be reduced and if necessary alternative forms of HRT used to allow body oestrogen levels to reduce gradually.

Implants are convenient and you do not have to remember to take or use oestrogen replacement on a regular basis. An implant may be used after hysterectomy, when you do not need progestogen. If you have a womb you will have to remember to take progestogen for 10–14 days of the cycle. A disadvantage of the implant is that the effects cannot be stopped quickly. When an implant is removed for the last time, you must continue to take a progestogen if you have a womb until withdrawal bleeding stops. The intrauterine progestogen-only system, Mirena, may be inserted into the womb to release 20mcg levonorgestrel per 24 hours because progestogen may be required for up to two years. This is an unofficial or 'off label' use of Mirena, which is usually used for contraception.

The male hormone, testosterone, is sometimes given by implant (dose range 25–100mg) with HRT to increase sexual drive, where libido is a significant problem, for example if you have had your ovaries removed before the menopause.

Other preparations

Other preparations that deliver oestrogen to the body include the **nasal spray** Aerodiol which contains 150mcg of estradiol (as estradiol hemihydrate) in each measured (metered) spray. Aerodiol can be used for menopausal symptoms. Initially one spray is used in each nostril at the same time each day, giving a total dose of 300mcg. The spray can be used cyclically for 21–28 days followed by a treatment-free period of two to seven days, or it can be used continuously without a break in treatment if appropriate. In both cases, progestogen must be taken for at least 12 days each cycle or month if you have not had a hysterectomy. The daily estradiol dose can be adjusted depending on symptom control to one to four sprays daily in divided doses, morning and evening. The need for continued treatment should be re-evaluated every six months.

When you spray Aerodiol into the nose, estradiol is absorbed through the lining of the nose directly into the body, bypassing the liver. It is best to clear your nose before you administer Aerodiol, for example if you have a runny nose, and to avoid blowing it or sniffing for 15 minutes afterwards (gentle wiping is fine). If your nose is severely blocked then you can use Aerodiol temporarily in the mouth, spraying between the cheek and the gum between the upper teeth, and using double the dose. If you use other nose drop or spray preparations, for example a corticosteroid or a decongestant for hayfever, then you should not use Aerodiol immediately afterwards. Local reactions to Aerodiol include tingling and sneezing; nose bleeds can occur.

The **vaginal ring** Menoring 50 is inserted into the vagina, where it releases estradiol: approximately 50mcg over 24 hours. It can be used for postmenopausal symptoms (especially those related to the bladder and vagina, such as dryness and soreness), if you have had a hysterectomy. Menoring 50 should remain in place for three months, after which time it is replaced by another ring. Progestogen should be taken for at least 12 days each month if you have not had a hysterectomy.

Vaginal creams, pessaries and rings

Local oestrogen cream or pessaries can be used in the vagina for dryness and soreness caused by the vaginal lining shrinking and drying (atrophy). Some women do not wish to use, or cannot take, systemic HRT (any form which raises hormone levels throughout the body) but need relief from symptoms such as a dry vagina and urinary problems. In such cases, oestrogen can be given locally to the vagina in the form of a low-dose cream, pessary (vaginal tablet) or ring. Both cream and pessaries are applied via applicators. The dose is inserted high into the vagina, preferably in the evening; detailed instructions are given with the products. Local irritation or itching may occur at the start of treatment.

Such preparations are also used before and after surgery, for example if you are having an operation for prolapse. Local oestrogen preparations include vaginal creams containing estriol or conjugated oestrogens, estriol or estradiol pessaries and an estradiol ring (see Table E).

These local preparations are applied to the vaginal lining, where HRT use is topical, that is applied to a body surface. Oestrogen is not likely to be absorbed significantly from the vagina into the body, particularly for the recommended short-term courses, for example up to three months with Ovestin or Vagifem, and so a progestogen is not needed. However, the Committee on Safety of Medicines (CSM) has stated that the effect on the endometrium of long-term or repeated use of local oestrogens in the vagina is largely uncertain. Long-term treatment should be stopped at least once a year and the need for ongoing treatment reviewed. If breakthrough bleeding or spotting occurs at any time while you are using local HRT discuss this with your doctor.

Table E: Oestrogen-only vaginal creams, pessaries and rings

Brand name	Vaginal preparation	Type of oestrogen
Ortho-Gynest	Cream	Estriol
	Pessaries	Estriol
Ovestin	Cream	Estriol
Premarin	Cream	Conjugated oestrogens
Vagifem	Vaginal tablets = pessaries	Estradiol
Estring	Ring	Estradiol

Estring is a vaginal ring made of silicone elastomer, which delivers a tiny dose of estradiol (7.5mcg in 24 hours), locally to the vagina to help vaginitis and urinary symptoms caused by atrophy and dryness after the menopause. The ring is placed high up in the vagina and is left in place for three months. It can be removed temporarily if needed, for example if it is uncomfortable during intercourse. The estradiol dose is small and it is not absorbed significantly into the bloodstream. Estring is not suitable for treating other post-menopausal symptoms or to prevent osteoporosis.

Progestogen preparations

Progesterone, or more usually a progestogen (synthetic equivalent), should always be used if you still have your uterus as it modifies some of the effects of oestrogen. Oestrogen replacement on its own, that is unopposed, can lead to a dose- and duration-dependent increase in endometrial problems. Oestrogen stimulates over-growth of the lining of the womb (hyperplasia), which can lead to cancerous changes. If you have not had a hysterectomy, unopposed oestrogen carries a substantial risk.

A progestogen given for 10–14 days out of 28 opposes the effect of oestrogen on the endometrial lining; newer combined HRT preparations have 14 days' worth of progestogen. This cyclical regimen usually leads to withdrawal bleeding towards the end of the progestogen course which replicates what the body was doing all through the woman's fertile years: oestrogen was present in the proliferative first half of the cycle, and then the ovary added proges-terone during the second half to protect the endometrium from excessive build-up and brought about a shedding (menstruation) at the correct time. Even so, the protective effects of progestogen can wear off with long-term use and hyperplasia may still develop, increasing the risk of endometrial cancer, despite regular with-drawal bleeding.

If you still have irregular periods, combined oestrogen and progestogen will help to make the cycle regular. A year after the menopause, a progestogen can be used on a continuous basis with oestrogen, both taken throughout the 28-day cycle. This avoids monthly bleeding, although irregular bleeding may occur within the first few months of using this type of HRT.

Dydrogesterone, norethisterone, norgestrel, levonorgestrel and **medroxyprogesterone** are commonly used in HRT preparations. Two progestogens, dydrogesterone and norethisterone, are also available as tablets (**Duphaston HRT** and **Micronor HRT** respectively). Either preparation can be added to any of the oestrogen-only preparations, described above, when the endometrium needs to be protected. Progesterone itself is not effective when taken by mouth. It is not used for HRT, although it is used in fertility treatment, for example.

Table F: Summary of advantages and disadvantages of types of HRT

HRT Type	Advantages	Disadvantages
Tablets: oestrogen-only or oestrogen + progestogen	Easy to start and stop	Remembering daily tablet taking Passes through the liver: unwanted effects troublesome but should settle with time (two to three months)
Skin patches	Easy and simple to use Unwanted effects lessened – bypasses liver	Local skin reactions Plaster residue Remembering to change patch
Skin gel	Easy to stop Unwanted effects lessened – bypasses liver	Messy to use every day Local skin reactions
Implants	No need to remember to take or change frequently Long-lasting Unwanted effects lessened – bypasses liver	Difficult to reverse HRT effect Has to be applied via surgical procedure Potential dosage difficulties (tachyphylaxis)
Local HRT: vaginal creams, pessaries, rings	Good for local vaginal problems Few unwanted systemic effects	Messy to use Oestrogen absorption unlikely to occur, but effects of long-term use uncertain

How long should you take HRT?

The duration of treatment depends on your reasons for taking HRT and you will need to discuss these with your doctor before starting it. Menopausal symptoms fade after some time but this varies from woman to woman. If you take HRT to relieve menopausal symptoms you could try a course for 6–12 months, then stop by reducing the dose gradually and see if troublesome symptoms return. You could restart if symptoms recur, but the increase in breast cancer risk begins within one to two years of starting treatment. In the UK, the average age when women start HRT is 50 years. Treatment is now mainly for menopausal symptoms and usually for two to three years. Once you have started HRT you must see your doctor for regular checks, yearly at least, to assess your health and the continuing need for treatment.

You should stop HRT immediately if any of the following occur:

- sudden severe pains in the chest
- sudden breathlessness or cough with blood spots in phlegm
- unexplained severe calf pain in one leg
- severe stomach pain
- unusual severe prolonged headache which seems to worsen
- sudden loss, or partial loss, of vision
- sudden disturbance of hearing or speech
- bad fainting attack or collapse, or unexplained seizure
- weakness or numbness suddenly affecting one side or one part of the body
- hepatitis or jaundice (yellowing of the skin or whites of the eyes)
- severe depression
- severe increase in blood pressure
- pregnancy.

When HRT must not be taken

Before you start HRT your doctor should take a complete personal and family medical history and carry out breast and pelvic examination. There are circumstances when HRT must not be taken, that is, it is contraindicated, including the following problems or situations:

- past, current or suspected breast cancer
- oestrogen-dependent cancers, for example, endometrial cancer
- undiagnosed vaginal bleeding
- untreated endometrial hyperplasia
- current untreated or past blood clots in the veins, for example, deep vein thrombosis in the legs or pelvis, blood clots on the lung (pulmonary embolism)

- active or recent cardiovascular disease, for example, angina, heart attack (myocardial infarction)
- active liver disease or where liver function tests have not returned to normal after a liver problem
- pregnancy
- breast-feeding.

These contraindications are included routinely in the information produced by manufacturers of HRT to warn doctors and women against using HRT in defined situations. In the UK, HRT use is not usually prescribed for women who have had breast cancer, but sometimes HRT is used in these situations because breast cancer treatment can trigger an early menopause and menopausal symptoms can be very troublesome. However, information from Sweden suggests that women who have had breast cancer and who then start HRT are at increased risk of having the disease again. The HABITS trial (Hormonal Replacement Therapy after Breast cancer – is it Safe?) started in 1997 and aimed to recruit 1,300 women who had had breast cancer previously and then to follow them up for an average of five years, but of the 434 enrolled initially, only 345 women continued with the trial. One group of women in the trial was given HRT and the other group was managed without hormone treatment, and researchers followed the progress of both groups. After an average follow-up of two years, 26 out of 174 women taking HRT had suffered a recurrence of the disease compared with only seven out of 171 women in the control group not taking hormonal treatment. The trial was stopped in December 2003 because the study had found that women with a history of breast cancer who then took HRT for menopausal symptoms were found to have an unacceptably high risk of developing breast cancer again, compared with women surviving breast cancer and not treated with hormones. However, a UK trial is also in progress because breast cancer survivors do need a strategy to cope with menopausal symptoms. If you have survived breast cancer and consider that your menopausal symptoms might be helped by HRT, then discuss the pros and cons with your specialist and GP. The CSM does not recommend HRT for women who have breast cancer or who have had it in the past. Furthermore, pharmaceutical companies that produce HRT will not be liable if anything untoward occurs while you use their products in situations for which their products are not recommended.

Cautious use of HRT

There are some situations in which it may be possible to use HRT but with caution and close monitoring. HRT may exacerbate (or aggravate) the following conditions, but women vary in their response to HRT treatment and so its use cannot be completely ruled out and must depend on individual circumstances:

- endometriosis, which may become worse as a result of the effect of oestrogen on the displaced endometrial tissues (reactivation)
- fibroids in the uterus, which are oestrogen-dependent, may increase in size but this can be monitored by pelvic examination and ultrasound
- a family history of or other risk factors for cardiovascular disease, for example, heart attack or angina
- diabetes mellitus, which may require restabilisation because blood glucose levels may change
- liver disease, depending on the cause and severity, although HRT that bypasses the liver may be acceptable
- risk factors for developing oestrogen-dependent breast cancer, for example, having a close relative with breast cancer
- history of endometrial hyperplasia, if adequate progestogen is used to oppose oestrogen treatment and there is no history of endometrial cancer
- otosclerosis, an unusual and possibly hereditary condition which produces hardening and fixation of the small bones in the middle ear, which may worsen
- gall bladder disease, which can be adversely affected by oestrogen owing to changes in bile composition with the increased risk of gall stones developing
- migraine or severe headaches, which may worsen
- systemic lupus erythematosus (autoimmune disease where body tissues are inflamed)
- epilepsy, because the condition may be exacerbated
- asthma, because the condition may be exacerbated

- high blood pressure, if the condition is treated adequately. HRT use if high blood pressure is untreated is associated with an increased risk of stroke
- blood clots in the deep veins, treated with warfarin to thin the blood.

Evidence for the benefits and risks of HRT

Around 20 million women worldwide in Western countries were using HRT at the end of the 1990s, many of whom were healthy women. Despite decades of HRT prescription the balance of risks and benefits for it remain uncertain. However, evidence has been accumulating about the potential for harm that can occur with the use of HRT.

Much of the evidence comes from the US Women's Health Initiative (WHI), which focuses on defining the risks and benefits of a number of strategies that might reduce long-term diseases such as heart disease, breast and bowel cancer, and fractures owing to osteoporosis in postmenopausal women. One trial looked at combined HRT in women who had not had a hysterectomy and the other investigated oestrogen-only HRT in hysterectomised women to assess whether HRT would reduce heart and circulatory disease in mostly healthy postmenopausal women. Results from these North American studies and also the UK Million Women Study (MWS) (see box) have largely confirmed the observations from many smaller trials, both randomised controlled and observational studies, which have been reported over the years since HRT started to become more widely used in the mid-1970s. In summary, HRT use has the potential to cause harm, which is a risk that must be balanced against its known benefits, and does not result in overall health gain in the longer term.

The WHI trials are particularly significant because they are double-blind randomised controlled trials conducted in healthy postmenopausal women where HRT use was compared with inactive or placebo treatment. A double-blind randomised controlled trial (the gold standard of clinical trials) is designed to eliminate error and bias in the study through the random assignment of the active treatment and placebo to trial participants.

Neither the doctors conducting the trial in different centres nor the participants know whether an active treatment or a placebo has been allocated (double-blind). In clinical trials some participants do drop out for a variety of reasons and the randomisation code may then be broken, but this is always reported in the trial results.

In the WHI trial of non-hysterectomised women, the most commonly used HRT in the USA – a continuous combined preparation containing conjugated oestrogens plus medroxyprogesterone acetate as the progestogen – was compared with women taking a matching placebo preparation. The average length of follow-up in the trial was just over five years. The trial was stopped early because overall the health risks, particularly harm from breast cancer, exceeded the benefits in healthy postmenopausal women. The WHI trial identified the absolute additional risks for 10,000 person years (an expression for measuring treatment time) as seven more cases of heart disease (near heart attacks or heart attacks particularly in the first year of HRT use), eight more strokes, eight more pulmonary embolism and eight more breast cancers. Some health benefits were identified, too, with six fewer colorectal cancers and five fewer hip fractures.

In contrast to the randomised controlled trial, the Million Women Study is an observational study and uses evidence collected from participants who are either established on treatment or not. Women who were invited to attend routine breast-screening mammography in the UK were also invited to complete a question-naire about HRT use and other health-related details. The study was conducted between 1996 and 2001: data were collected on over 1 million women. In this group of women 50 per cent had used HRT at some time. One-third of the women were current users with a mean duration on HRT of nearly six years. The study found that current users of HRT, particularly combined HRT, were more likely to have breast cancer and die from it than women who had never used HRT. Estimates from the MWS suggest that six additional cases of breast cancer occur with five years' use and 19 additional cases with ten years' use in 1,000 women taking combined HRT. The risk of breast cancer therefore increases the longer combined HRT is used over time. While this type of study can identify factors that influence disease outcomes, it can be subject to bias. Since its publication, menopause experts have questioned the

Summary of the Women's Health Initiative trials (WHI) and the Million Women Study (MWS)

Study elements	Women's Health Initiative (USA)	Women's Health Initiative (USA)	Million Women Study (UK)
Objective	To assess major health benefits and risks of most commonly used combined HRT	To assess major health benefits and risks of most commonly used oestrogen-only preparation (Premarin)	To investigate the relation between various patterns of use of HRT and breast cancer incidence (occurrence) and death
Type of trial	Double-blind randomised controlled trial	Double-blind randomised controlled trial	Observational
Study population	16,608 postmenopausal women aged 50–79 years eligible for a trial of combined HRT (non-hysterectomised)	10,739 postmenopausal hysterectomised women aged 50–79 years eligible for a trial of oestrogen-only HRT	1,084,110 women aged 50–64 years (not registered as having had cancer) invited to attend the national breast screening programme
Study treatment	Conjugated oestrogens 625mcg + progestogen as medroxyprogesterone acetate 2.5mg in one tablet taken daily (8,506 women) or daily placebo (8,102 women)	Conjugated oestrogens 625mcg in one tablet daily (5,310 women) or daily placebo (5,429 women)	Reported use of all types of HRT – if ever used, current use, past use and dates, total duration of use, name of most recent HRT taken and its duration of use – plus reported non-users of HRT
Study outcome measures	Effect of HRT on heart disease, hip fracture, breast cancer and on overall health	Effect of HRT on heart disease, hip fracture, breast cancer and on overall health	Estimate of numbers of women who may develop breast cancer and die from it
Duration of trial	Average follow-up 5.2 years	Average follow-up 6.8 years	Average follow-up for cancer incidence 2.6 years; average follow-up for deaths 4.1 years
Conclusion	Long-term use of combined HRT does not improve health by preventing heart disease in postmenopausal women. Risk of fractures and of developing colorectal cancer decreases with HRT use but these benefits are offset by increases in risk of breast cancer, heart disease, stroke and pulmonary embolism	Oestrogen-only HRT increases the risk of stroke, but decreases the risk of hip fractures and does not affect heart disease. A possible reduction in breast cancer risk occurred but more information is needed. Oestrogen-only HRT is not recommended for preventing long-term health problems in postmenopausal women	Current and recent users of HRT are at increased risk of developing breast cancer and of dying from the disease. The effect is greater for combined HRT than for other types of HRT

conclusions of the MWS, even though the results are similar to the WHI trial, and both studies have been reviewed by the CSM.

The oestrogen-only HRT component of the US WHI in hysterectomised women compared conjugated oestrogens with placebo and reported results more recently. It found that oestrogen-only HRT increased the risk of stroke but did not affect the risk of heart disease. Oestrogen-only HRT reduced the risk of hip and other fractures as expected, but surprisingly the study found a non-significant reduction in breast cancer risk over almost seven years of use. This result contradicts most other observational studies, including the MWS, which found a modest increase in breast cancer risk with oestrogen-only HRT, although much less so than for combined HRT. Further investigations on the impact of oestrogen-only HRT on the risk of breast cancer will be needed.

HRT and breast cancer risk

In 2003 the CSM published summaries of two studies, the observational UK Million Women Study and the Women's Health Initiative, which looked at the long-term safety of HRT. Further guidance was published by the CSM in December 2003 and is endorsed by similar medicines regulatory authorities across Europe and the USA (*www.mhra.gov.uk*; *www.emea.eu.int*; *www.fda.gov*).

The guidance is summarised as follows.

- Studies confirm that the risk of breast cancer increases with HRT use.
- The increase in risk starts within one to two years of starting any type of HRT.
- The longer HRT is used, the higher the risk of breast cancer.
- The risk starts to decline when HRT is stopped, and five years after a woman stops taking it, the risk reaches the same level as in women who have never taken HRT.
- Women using combined HRT (oestrogen and progestogen) have a higher risk of developing breast cancer than women using oestrogen-only HRT.
- Tibolone, the synthetic HRT preparation with oestrogenic and progestogenic activity, also increases the risk of breast cancer, but the risk is not as high as with combined HRT.

When the cancer risk is assessed for women aged 50–65 years, the extra number of breast cancer cases per 1,000 HRT users for **combined HRT** is estimated as six with five years' use, and 19 with ten years' use. For **oestrogen-only HRT**, the extra number of breast cancer cases is fewer: around one additional case for five years' use, and five for ten years' use. Since the CSM guidance in December 2003, new evidence from the Women's Health Initiative trial suggests that oestrogen-only HRT may not be associated with an increased risk of breast cancer, although those involved in the trial say that this requires further investigation because the results were not statistically significant. These results for oestrogen-only HRT seem to contradict those from many observational studies, including the UK Million Women Study. Whether the CSM guidance will be modified in the light of the latest results from the Women's Health Initiative remains a point of conjecture. In the meantime most doctors are likely to follow the CSM guidance, although some specialists do not support the government's line.

Clearly, women who have never used HRT also develop breast cancer. The CSM has calculated that for women aged 50 years who do not use HRT, about 32 in every 1,000 will be diagnosed with breast cancer by the time they reach the age of 65 years. There is an additional risk of developing breast cancer while taking HRT. This risk has to be carefully weighed against benefits of taking HRT for controlling menopausal and postmenopausal symptoms. The extra number of cases attributed to HRT is small, particularly when compared with the health risks associated with smoking or obesity.

If you take HRT, including oestrogen-only or tibolone, regular review is essential. Be 'breast aware' – check regularly, note any changes that occur including changes to the skin and nipples and the appearance of lumps, and discuss promptly any concerns with your doctor. When you are 50 years or over you can attend breast screening (see Chapter 9 for details).

Other cancer risks with HRT

Endometrial cancer
As mentioned previously, oestrogen stimulates the uterus lining, resulting in abnormal growth or endometrial hyperplasia, which can lead to the development of endometrial disease including cancer. The increased risk of endometrial cancer occurs if you take

oestrogen on its own and have not had a hysterectomy. Taking a progestogen for 12–14 days each month continuously lowers the risk and should largely counteract this problem.

The safety of using local HRT as an oestrogen cream or pessaries in the vagina long term or as repeated courses is largely uncertain. Oestrogen can be absorbed from the vagina into the body and therefore influence endometrial growth, but the extent to which this happens is unknown. In the UK, it appears that most local oestrogen preparations are used without the addition of progestogen systemically.

Any abnormal vaginal bleeding, such as heavy or irregular bleeding or bleeding regularly after sex, that occurs some months after starting HRT, including local use, should be discussed with your doctor. Breakthrough bleeding or spotting is fairly common during the first few months of starting HRT, but if it continues for longer or starts after you have been taking HRT for some time or continues after you have stopped HRT then tell your doctor.

Ovarian cancer

There is a slightly increased risk of ovarian cancer if you take **oestrogen-only HRT**. The extra number of ovarian cancer cases in 1,000 oestrogen-only HRT users is around one with five years' use and three with ten years' use compared with non-HRT users among women aged 50–69 years. The additional risk is very small for short-term use of HRT. The risks of developing ovarian cancer with combined HRT (oestrogen and progestogen) are unclear at present and further research is needed.

HRT and the risk of abnormal blood clots

The risk of abnormal blood clots developing in the deep veins within the body increases with HRT, especially in the first year of treatment. Known as venous thromboembolism (VTE), the term covers deep vein thrombosis (DVT) and pulmonary embolism (PE), but exactly how HRT increases this risk is not exactly clear. It appears that some factors in blood that affect normal clotting mechanisms alter with the menopause and that HRT increases certain body chemicals in the blood coagulation cascade process within blood vessels. The overall effect is an increased risk of blood clots forming which have the potential to cause harm.

Around three women in 1,000 women not taking HRT in their 50s will have a VTE over a five-year period. When women take HRT, for those aged 50–59 years the extra number of VTE cases is estimated as four, and for women aged 60–69 years the extra number of cases is nine per 1,000 HRT users over a five-year period. The risks are greater if you:

- have a personal or strong family history of venous thrombo-embolism, severe and extensive varicose veins or heart failure
- have had a recent heart attack
- are overweight
- are of an advanced age
- are undergoing major trauma or surgery
- have to lie in bed for some time because of an accident or a prolonged illness
- travel on a long-haul flight (over six hours).

If you are already on anticoagulant treatment for thinning the blood, such as warfarin, then you can start HRT, as the risk of VTE with hormonal treatment should be minimised.

All types of HRT preparation seem to increase the risk of VTE, although HRT which bypasses the liver may be less of a problem. The increased risk of VTE disappears rapidly on stopping HRT treatment.

HRT and surgery

If you have an operation booked for a particular date you will need to discuss whether or not you should stop HRT beforehand. Doctors advise that hormonal treatment, HRT or the combined oral contraceptive pill (but not the progestogen-only pill) should be stopped four weeks before surgery. Alternatively, you could continue hormonal treatment through the period of hospitalisation providing you receive standard measures to prevent the development of blood clots. Measures include treatment to thin the blood, for example with heparin and by wearing compression stockings. These measures should also cover you if you need emergency surgery while taking HRT. If you suspend hormonal treatments, these can be restarted once you are fully active again.

HRT and stroke

HRT slightly increases the risk of a user having a stroke. As you grow older the risk of stroke increases, and when you are in your 50s, it is estimated that about three in 1,000 women not using HRT will have a stroke in any five-year period. For women aged 50–59 years, one extra stroke occurs for every 1,000 women using HRT for five years. For women in their 60s not using HRT about 11 in 1,000 will have a stroke over a five-year period compared with about 15 who use HRT for five years. Therefore, the number of extra strokes is four for women aged 60–69 for every 1,000 women using HRT over a five-year period. Early warning signs of a stroke include unusual migraine-type headaches or unusual fainting or temporary weakness in the arms or legs. You should see your doctor if any of these problems occur.

Summary of HRT use

In summary, HRT provides good relief when menopausal symptoms, particularly hot flushes and night sweats, threaten to disrupt your life. It is preferable to use HRT for the short term, although the CSM has not defined short-term use. Treatment should be with the most convenient preparation for you at the lowest effective dose and be reviewed at least once a year by your doctor. If you have experienced a premature menopause, HRT can be used for relieving symptoms and for preventing osteoporosis up to the age of 50 years, provided you have regular reviews. HRT is no longer recommended if you are healthy with no troublesome menopausal or postmenopausal symptoms.

Chapter 6

Alternatives to HRT

In the Western world the menopause is a major event in a woman's life, often associated with its own distinct symptoms and diseases (see Chapter 2 for how the experience of menopause differs across cultures). There are huge individual differences in the symptoms women have and the long-term health risks that are consequences of it. In addition, the treatment options that women can consider using are wide-ranging. Many women are choosing to avoid hormone replacement therapy (HRT, see box below), certainly until the effects and safety of oestrogen and progestogens become clearer. Instead they are opting for complementary and alternative therapies and lifestyle changes. Alternative approaches to the menopause can offer a variety of treatment options, to women who either cannot take HRT or who would prefer to avoid it, for both symptom relief and for long-term health protection.

Reasons why some women avoid using HRT

Not all women use HRT to alleviate the symptoms of the menopause. The reasons they avoid it include:

- other health problems that preclude the use of HRT
- concern about the long-term risks of HRT
- fear of the side-effects of HRT
- concern that HRT interferes with nature
- worries over continued vaginal bleeding
- desire to be in control of one's own health
- the inadequacy of the information available
- conflicting or confusing advice.

Alternative approaches to menopause treatment fall into four groups:

- complementary medicine
- dietary changes
- lifestyle changes
- alternative prescribed medication.

Complementary medicine and therapies

Complementary and alternative medicine (CAM) is more popular in the UK today than ever before, with an estimated 4–5 million people seeing a complementary therapist each year. The reasons for the increase in acceptance and use of such therapies are both negative (such as disillusionment with certain aspects of conventional medicine) and positive (the fact that so many people claim to have benefited from them). *The Which? Guide to Complementary Therapies* discusses the subject of CAM in great detail.

For women going through the menopause, CAM is generally used to help relieve short-term symptoms; it is unlikely to have any effect on the long-term consequences, except by helping with lifestyle changes that have an impact on health into old age, such as weight control and smoking.

Research suggests that most people tend to use CAM alongside conventional medicine, rather than as an alternative to it. This is borne out in the case of menopause too: one study in 2001 in the UK showed that 21 per cent of menopausal women used CAM alone but 25 per cent used a combination of it and HRT.

Drawbacks of CAM
Just as HRT is given under medical supervision because of the safety issues associated with it (see Chapter 5), anyone using CAM needs to understand that there is also the potential for harm, either because the treatment is not effective or because there are possible risks and side-effects associated with the treatment itself. Some of the therapies and products used in CAM may not have been studied adequately for us to be certain of their benefits or to highlight possible side-effects.

CAM lacks a research tradition and also a research infrastructure. Although the situation is changing, funding for research into such treatments is generally quite limited compared with the amount spent by the pharmaceutical industry on conventional drugs.

This lack of adequate research clearly works against CAM. There may well be complementary treatments that are effective to treat menopause problems and practitioners who from their own experience and expertise know that these treatments do work, but without properly conducted studies, these benefits cannot be proven.

As a result, some conventional doctors have been sceptical of CAM. However, because many women, even those with unpleasant menopausal symptoms, are opting to avoid HRT, it is becoming increasingly important that practitioners and women are aware of the treatment choices available.

Choosing a therapy and therapist

Deciding whether to opt for CAM, and choosing which therapy is best for you, can be daunting, given the number of therapies available and the differences between them.

Over 200 different complementary therapies are in existence. Some of them, such as acupuncture, chiropractic, herbal medicine, homeopathy and osteopathy, are better known and more commonly used than others. The therapies considered to be most beneficial for the relief of short-term menopausal symptoms are herbal medicine, homeopathy, nutritional therapy and relaxation therapy.

If you wish to try CAM, you must find a well-trained, reputable practitioner. It is vital that you check out the therapist's credentials, and it is also important to choose a practitioner you feel comfortable with. Personal recommendation can be a good way of finding such a therapist, but not always. If you have decided what therapy you want to try, then you could contact the relevant registering body (or bodies), as some of them will supply you with a list of qualified practitioners in your area. You could also take advice from your GP, but he or she may be unenthusiastic about CAM as a whole or may be no better informed about it than you are. Many well-qualified practitioners advertise in *Yellow Pages*, but bear in mind that anyone can be listed. It is inadvisable, however, to look for therapists at natural healing fairs and festivals, in advertisements displayed in shop windows, or via a mail-shot through your door. Also, regard anyone who approaches you directly, in person or by phone or email, with suspicion: reputable practitioners do not hawk for business.

Whatever way you find a therapist, always check his or her qualifications with the organisation to which he or she claims to belong. However, even membership of a body is no guarantee of quality and good practice – you need to be sure that the organisation itself is reputable.

The best organisations will have the following safeguards:

- a set of validated, and accredited, educational and training standards
- a code of practice and ethics
- a complaints procedure
- disciplinary procedures
- a requirement for indemnity insurance.

For each of the therapies discussed below, the main organisations are named (and their contact details can be found at the back of the book). In addition to them there are umbrella bodies, which primarily represent the interests of practitioners, which may not necessarily be those of consumers. There are two main organisations.

The British Complementary Medicine Association (BCMA)★ claims to represent about 25,000 practitioners in 67 organisations covering 30 therapies. It is the organisations – and not the individuals who belong to them – that pay to be on the register that the BCMA runs. Members of the public can contact the BCMA either to check on the qualifications of a practitioner or to a find a qualified therapist in a particular field who practises in their area.

The Institute of Complementary Medicine (ICM)★ provides information to the public about complementary practitioners. It claims to represent about 2,000 therapists in nearly 800 organisations covering 18 therapies on its British Register of Complementary Practitioners (BRCP).

Herbal medicine

Herbal medicine is the use of plants to treat disease and promote good health. Many herbs are the precursors to modern drugs: examples include the heart medication digoxin that comes from foxgloves, and salicylic acid (similar to aspirin) that is derived from meadow sweet. About a quarter of all pharmaceutical preparations contain an active plant ingredient. However, herbalists rarely isolate the active ingredient from the plant, using the whole plant instead, believing the remedy works through a delicate balance of all the constituents in the plant. It is thought that these work together to enhance its action, to make it safe and minimise side-effects.

Many people think that herbal remedies are 'natural' and therefore harmless. However, some herbs may contain potent chemicals and should be used with caution. As the active ingredient in many preparations is unknown, women with a history of other health problems such as breast cancer or thrombosis, or women on other medicines should not use herbal remedies without discussion first with a healthcare practitioner. There are a number of known drug-herb interactions and caution is needed with mixing herbs and pharmaceutical drugs. Always buy reputable, well-known brands and tell your practitioner what you are taking.

In the UK, there are Western herbalists (who use remedies derived solely from plant sources), Chinese herbalists (who mainly use remedies from the Far East and who include in their preparations ingredients derived from plant, animal and mineral sources) and Ayurvedic practitioners (who mainly use remedies from India, sourced from plants and minerals). The herbal remedies discussed below are all Western because there is more evidence about their suitability for relieving menopause-related symptoms than there is for the other two types.

In the UK, anyone can set themselves up as a herbalist but, although most herbalists are not medically trained, the majority undergo extensive training. To choose a qualified Western herbalist, contact the National Institute of Medical Herbalists (NIMH)★.

Black cohosh
A herb native to Eastern North America, black cohosh (Cimicifuga) is traditionally used by native Americans for a variety of gynaecological complaints including hot flushes and sweats, menopausal anxiety and depression. A review in 1998 of a number of clinical studies of a standardised extract of black cohosh (Remifemin) reported some improvement of flushes, insomnia and low mood. However, a study in 2002 showed that black cohosh did not

improve menopause symptoms. No drug interactions have been reported in the medical literature but a few side-effects such as nausea, vomiting, headaches, breast tenderness and weight gain have been noticed in trials. A daily dose of 40–80mg is used, with a recommended duration of treatment no longer than six months.

Other herbs
Other herbal remedies often recommended by CAM practitioners for the menopause include St John's Wort, valerian, sage, chaste tree, dong quai, ginseng, ginko biloba, kava, garlic and feverfew. Scientific data on the effectiveness of these is limited, and there is concern about side-effects or drug interactions.

Oil of evening primrose
Oil of evening primrose is a popular supplement taken by many women. It does not seem to have any effect on menopausal flushes and sweats but it can be helpful in improving breast tenderness and premenstrual symptoms.

Homeopathy

There is no scientific proof that homeopathy is effective in treating menopausal symptoms, but anecdotal reports suggest that it is helpful. Homeopathy is one of the most widely accepted therapies and is sometimes available on the NHS.

Homeopathy uses remedies derived from plant, mineral and occasionally animal sources that are diluted many, many times over. It has been questioned whether any molecules of the original substance actually remain. Between each dilution, the mixture is shaken vigorously (known as sucussion) so that the cure leaves its 'footprint' in the solution.

Many homeopaths practise what is called classical homeopathy, that is, they claim to treat each patient as an individual and attempt to identify the ideal remedy for that person's general make-up or constitution. In this type of homeopathy, diseases are not diagnosed in the same way as those diagnosed by conventional doctors, although the homeopath will want to know the conventional diagnosis too. The remedy selected is based only partly on your symptoms and also takes into account your constitutional characteristics and emotional responses. There are also homeopaths who prescribe on the basis of a conventional medical diagnosis or symptoms only. These tend to be conventionally trained doctors.

Homeopathic remedies are available as tinctures, lactose-based tablets, pills, granules and powders to be taken by mouth, and some also come as creams or ointments to be applied directly to the skin.

Anyone can set himself or herself up as a homeopath. But, while most homeopaths in the UK are not medically trained, the majority have had extensive training. To find a properly qualified lay homeopath, contact the Society of Homoeopaths*.

Homeopathic remedies are also now widely available in pharmacies and health food shops to purchase for self-treatment. While this is convenient, the drawback with off-the-shelf remedies is that they are not specifically tailored to the individual and picking a remedy can be a bit hit-and-miss.

Nutritional therapy

Nutritional therapy, or nutritional medicine, is the use of diet and nutritional supplements as the main treatment for disease. In the case of menopause-related symptoms, a soya-rich diet has been shown to be effective. It is discussed in detail under Dietary changes.

Anyone can call him- or herself a nutritional therapist, even if he or she has had only minimal training. The British Association of Nutritional Therapists (BANT)* holds a register of about 200 therapists.

Relaxation therapy

True relaxation occurs when the mind is still, the muscles deeply relaxed and the breathing slow and regular. There are several techniques that can help you relax this way, such as meditation, deep breathing and muscle relaxation, and all of them can be mastered quite easily with a little practice.

Relaxation techniques and meditation are used by a wide range of people, for many different reasons. Some people meditate for spiritual reasons, others to relieve stress and improve well-being. Relaxation techniques and meditation are also used to treat specific conditions, particularly those that are triggered or made worse by stress, such as high blood pressure, anxiety, insomnia, phobias and menstrual and menopausal problems. There is promising evidence from trials looking at relaxation for menopausal symptoms (see 'Stress', below).

In the UK, three types of meditation are widely practised. Transcendental meditation (TM)★, which is practised by around 200,000 people in the UK, is used predominantly to relieve stress. Buddhist meditation practices involve developing awareness of breathing and of positive feelings for all living beings, in an attempt to achieve inner peace and calm. The Friends of the Western Buddhist Order (FWBO)★ runs meditation classes around the UK. Vedic mantra meditation, as taught by the School of Meditation★ in London, is a technique that allows the attention to rest on a simple sound to which you attach no attitude or emotions. This gives access to the deeper, still part of the mind.

Dietary changes

Many of the dietary changes ideally need to be adopted in early life to create good habits and maximise the benefits later in life (see Chapter 7). However, many women find that taking steps to alter their eating habits helps alleviate some of the symptoms of the menopause.

Caffeine

Caffeine, which is present in chocolate and cola as well as tea and coffee, can make flushes worse. It is also a diuretic and can add to the urinary problems (such as frequency, urgency to get to a toilet and incontinence) that some women begin to experience at the menopause. Having caffeine at night affects the ability of some women to go to sleep, and increases the likelihood of their getting up during the night to pass urine. Caffeine has also been shown to have a detrimental effect on bone density but not when it is incorporated into a high-calcium diet. Try drinking water and caffeine-free drinks as an alternative. There are many interesting caffeine-free teas available, but for some women merely having hot drinks can bring on a flush.

Alternatives to HRT

	Complementary therapies	Dietary changes and supplements	Lifestyle changes	Pharmacological alternatives and OTC products
Vasomotor symptoms	Stress-reducing therapies Herbalism	Phytoestrogens Multivitamins/ minerals Reduce caffeine, alcohol and spicy food	Reduce stress Avoid trigger factors Avoid smoking Avoid heat Exercise	Antidepressants
Mood swings	Stress-reducing/ nutritional therapies Herbalism	Oil of evening primrose (PMS)	Exercise support groups	Antidepressants
Vaginal/ urinary symptoms	Aromatherapy Herbalism	Phytoestrogens	Pelvic exercises Regular intercourse Reduce caffeine	Long-acting vaginal moisturisers Simple lubricants
Insomnia	Stress-reducing therapies Herbalism	Reduce caffeine	Exercise Relaxation techniques	Night sedation
Heart disease	Therapies to help with lifestyle changes Nutritional therapies	Reduce cholesterol Moderate alcohol Take vitamin/ mineral supplements	Exercise Reduce weight, smoking and stress	Blood pressure- and cholesterol- reducing medication
Osteoporosis	Therapies to help with lifestyle changes Nutritional therapies	Calcium/ Vitamin D Reduce sodium, animal protein, alcohol, caffeine	Exercise Reduce smoking	Bisphosphonates Raloxifene

Salt

It has been known for many years that there is a connection between high levels of salt intake and loss of calcium through urine: the more salt a woman has the more calcium she loses. This may be significant if the calcium intake is limited (see Chapter 7). An average salt intake of 9g/day was not shown to constitute a risk for bones. A high-protein diet, generally in the form of animal protein, also raises urinary calcium loss and probably adds to the sodium effect. However, in older women, protein in the diet is essential to maintain the microstructure of the bone. High phosphorus intake has also been linked to increased urinary calcium loss. Phosphorus is present in fizzy drinks and it is probably a more significant risk factor in young people if they are drinking canned drinks and no milk.

Alcohol

Alcohol can make flushes worse. The effect of alcohol on the risk of fracture is puzzling: moderate alcohol intake (ten to 14 units per week, where a unit is a glass of wine or half a pint of beer) appears to increase bone density, but there is a weak positive association with fracture risk. However, heavy drinkers are more likely to smoke and have poor diets, which in turn will increase their risk of osteoporosis. Excessive amounts of alcohol raise the blood pressure, which in the long term is harmful.

Dietary supplements

There has been a massive rise in the use of food supplements and other nutrients over the past few years. This may in part be due to the concern over side-effects and unwanted reactions of prescriptions drugs, including HRT. Undoubtedly diet can influence and even improve one's chances of recovering from a disease (for example, people with coeliac disease eating wheat-free diets). Many menopausal women regularly use dietary supplements to reduce menopause symptoms and to generally improve good health. A study in 2002 in the UK showed that among women over 60 years of age, 65 per cent used foods supplements, believing that they contributed to good health. The number of dietary supplements has mushroomed over the past five years but knowledge about the effects of these products on the menopause is still very limited. It is hoped that this will change before too long.

The effect of diet on the menopause has been studied for a long time. Over recent years the use of nutraceuticals has been of special interest to scientists. These are substances that are derived from food, plant or other natural origin and have therapeutic properties.

They are nutrients that can influence and improve many disease processes in the body, and include vitamins and minerals.

Vitamins and minerals

Studies of vitamins and minerals and menopausal symptoms date back to the 1940s. Some anecdotal evidence suggests that multivitamin and mineral supplements can reduce flushes, but their effect may be partly dependent on the quality of the individual woman's diet. Many such preparations are available and targeted at menopausal women.

Vitamin E is said to reduce vasomotor symptoms, so many nutritional therapists recommend that menopausal women take the vitamin in the form of a supplement, with apparent success.

Despite dietary supplements becoming increasingly popular, it is worrying that users seldom associate side-effects with supplement use. Most people get information about supplements from their friends or family, the media and magazines – and rarely from health professionals – so they may not have an accurate impression of them.

Natural progesterone creams

Skin creams containing natural progesterone have been available over the counter and via mail order for about twenty years. They are unlicensed and sold under the umbrella of a dietary supplement. This 'natural' progesterone is extracted from plant sources, mainly yams and soya, and is structurally identical to the body's own progesterone. The evidence to support their use is limited; however, one study did report an improvement in flushes and sweats. They have no effect on bones, so they should not be used for the prevention or treatment of osteoporosis. The absorption of the progesterone from the cream is limited. It should not be used in HRT instead of progestogen, as it does not offer the protection the endometrium needs. However, some women do report improvements in menopausal symptoms and feelings of well-being when using the cream, and an ongoing trial will confirm whether this is a true response to the treatment or not.

Phytoestrogens

In recent years, soya and phytoestrogens (see also Chapter 10) have created much interest among the public and pharmaceutical industry in their attempt to identify effective alternatives to HRT. Phytoestrogens are compounds that are found in plants to differing degrees. They are structurally similar to estradiol and may mimic its action in the body. However, they are much weaker than the body's own natural oestrogen. There are many different types of phyto-estrogens but it is the isoflavones such as genistein and lignans that are thought to be particularly significant at the menopause. Isoflavones are found in legumes and soya bean, and lignans are found in seed oils, cereals, fruit and vegetables. Phytoestrogens need to be digested and metabolised in the gut, so that the active compounds can be absorbed into the body. The degree to which individuals can metabolise, absorb and benefit from phytoestrogens varies.

Diet is thought to be one factor that helps explain the cultural differences in the menopause experience (see Chapter 2). Asian women experience fewer menopausal symptoms than Western women and their traditional diets contain high levels of phyto-estrogens – about 200mg daily compared with less than 5mg daily in a Western diet.

To take one example, the traditional Japanese diet is rich in soya. It does not seem to be a coincidence that there is no word in Japanese for the menopausal hot flush – the symptom does not seem to exist. Moreover, the Japanese have a lower risk of heart disease, osteoporosis and cancers of the ovary, breast, endometrium, prostate and colon. Furthermore, women with breast cancer in Japan tend to have a better outcome than those with breast cancer in the USA or the UK.

The evidence that phytoestrogens reduce menopausal symptoms is confusing. Some studies have shown that they do reduce and improve flushes, while others have not shown this. Most of the studies have been small and fairly short term. However, because phytoestrogens have a very weak oestrogen effect and any improvements may not show up for at least three months, it may simply be that many of the studies had not gone on for long enough to show the benefits. Most studies have used doses of 40–80mg of isoflavones daily. Even though the results of the different studies are not consistent, none of the studies has shown any problematic side-effects from phytoestrogens.

Small studies of phytoestrogens have shown some improvement in vaginal symptoms of dryness and discomfort with intercourse.

Some useful recipes

Menopause muesli

1lb   jumbo oats
4oz   oat bran
4oz   wheat flakes
4oz   raisins
4oz   chopped dried apricots
4oz   chopped dried dates
2oz   dried banana flakes
2oz   sunflower seeds
2oz   pumpkin seeds
2oz   toasted sesame seeds
2oz   linseeds

Mix all the ingredients together. Store it in an airtight container and serve with soya milk.

Menopause cake

4oz   soya flour
4oz   wholemeal flour
4oz   rolled oats
4oz   linseeds
2oz   sunflower seeds
2oz   pumpkin seeds
2oz   sesame seeds
2oz   flaked almonds
2 pieces of stem ginger, finely chopped
8oz   raisins
Half teaspoon of nutmeg, cinnamon and ground ginger
15fl oz soya milk
1 tablespoon of malt extract

Put all the dry ingredients in a mixing bowl. Add the soya milk and malt extract, mix well and leave for about 30 minutes to soak. Heat the oven to 190°C/375°F/gas mark 5. Line a small loaf tin with baking parchment. Spoon the mixture into the tin and bake for 90 minutes. Test with a skewer. Turn out and cool on a wire rack. Eat with soya spread.

There are debates about the effects of phytoestrogens on the cardio-vascular system and blood pressure.

Many dietary supplements of phytoestrogens are available, as many women would find it impossible to alter their diets to such a degree to incorporate sufficient levels of them. It is possible to buy a bread that is high in phytoestrogens (it is made from soya flour and contains linseeds). It has been reported that four slices a day help reduce flushes. Some supermarkets stock dairy products made from soya that contain guaranteed amounts of phytoestrogens. Recipes have been devised for muesli and a cake (see page 101) that have ingredients packed with phytoestrogens. However, be aware of the calories that these products contain, as weight often becomes a concern for women at the menopause.

It is not known whether taking phytoestrogens as part of a Western diet will produce the same effects as they do in a traditional Asian diet. Any differences in the incidence of disease in other cultures (such as a lower breast cancer risk in Japan), which are in part due to diet, are likely to be the result of a lifetime's exposure to the diet.

There remain many gaps in our knowledge and understanding of the effects of phytoestrogens, but they are certainly worthy of more research.

Lifestyle changes

Women experiencing the menopause can help alleviate their symptoms by making certain changes to their lifestyle.

Minimising triggers of hot flushes

It is well recognised that there are 'trigger' factors that have an impact on some menopausal symptoms, making them worse. Hot flushes can be triggered by alcohol, caffeine, smoking, hot or spicy food or drinks, together with a hot environment, and stress, so if flushing and night sweating are an inconvenient or distressing problem, try avoiding these as much as possible. You may need to review the way you dress. Try wearing layers that can be easily removed and then replaced, such as a light cardigan over a shirt, instead of a single jumper. Good ventilation, minimal heating and light bed linen may help symptoms become more bearable but may be unpopular with partners, family and colleagues. Try to encourage the family to wear warmer clothes, so that you can keep the house cooler. Keep a small battery-powered fan in your handbag or pocket for when you are on the move.

Smoking

It is well worth highlighting some of the effects of smoking at the menopause. As mentioned earlier, smokers tend to have a slightly earlier menopause than non-smokers. Smoking is a trigger factor for hot flushes. For women on HRT, it appears that smoking may cancel out the effect of oral oestrogen. This means that the HRT may not have the desired beneficial effect on flushes and will also have a reduced effect on the bones and urinary and vaginal symptoms. Smoking is associated with reduced bone formation: smokers and past smokers have lower bone densities than non-smokers. This is probably because of the toxic effect of nicotine on osteoblasts (cells that lay down new bone and strengthen it with calcium).

Stress

Encouraging women to reassess their priorities in life to reduce unnecessary stress may help alleviate some symptoms. Stress can contribute to flushes and sweats, anxiety, low mood and poor sleep. Complementary therapies (see 'Complementary medicine and therapies', above) can help with stress relief and increase relaxation.

For many women, the menopause coincides with other stressful events in their lives. Often menopausal women are caught between pressures from both the older and younger generations. These issues may result from having adolescent children, children leaving home or even the responsibility of grandchildren; ageing parents or the loss of a parent; marriage or other relationship problems; financial difficulties and worries about pensions; and changes in work and home responsibilities. Just getting older, with all the body changes that occur, can be distressing for some women. Most of the time there are no easy answers, so it is important to find opportunities to relax, forget the pressures and perhaps pamper yourself. These could include taking a long bath, reading a book, meeting a friend or pursuing an interest or hobby.

Some women find that it is necessary to reduce the pressures of daily living. Others find that their home and work responsibilities have dwindled resulting in them feeling bored or unwanted. Finding new roles or a job can be daunting. However, there are many courses available to help with retraining, updating skills (such as IT skills) or opportunities to do charitable work. Check out local papers, libraries and colleges for ideas.

In other cultures where extended families are common, support is then close at hand. However in the Western world, where we tend to live in small nuclear units, many women feel alone. Studies have highlighted the value of support groups for menopausal women in helping them overcome the feeling of isolation or alienation. If you can get together with other menopausal women to meet regularly, it can help you realise that many others go through experiences that you thought were unique to you. If such a group does not exist in your area, then speak to the nurse at your local GP practice, as it may be possible to set one up. An occupational health nurse at work may be helpful; otherwise it might be possible to confide in a friend. If the issues are very distressing, then speak to your GP. Referral to a counsellor may be appropriate.

Exercise

Exercise is tremendously important for many reasons throughout life and this is particularly true at the time of the menopause. It is helpful for so many things:

- women who exercise regularly have fewer hot flushes and sweats
- exercise enhances mood, and regular exercise can reduce feelings of depression and improve feelings of well-being
- generally, people who exercise sleep better
- regular exercise, alongside a sensible eating regimen can help to control weight
- exercise helps to protect the bones from increased bone loss at and after the menopause
- joining a gym or a rambling club to exercise can help provide social opportunities
- regular exercise can help reduce blood pressure and reduce the risk of heart disease.

Women should generally exercise for at least 30 minutes three or four times a week. It may be necessary for you to build up to these gradually and you may have to be imaginative to find ways of making these sessions fit in with what could be an already busy life. Running a home alongside a job is often very busy but for many women it does not include sufficient exercise. So make the most of all exercise opportunities such as taking the stairs instead of a lift, avoiding using a car for short trips, and planning and allocating specific, realistic amounts of time for exercise.

Pelvic floor exercises

Pelvic floor exercises (see also Chapter 8) can be beneficial for women at and after the menopause to help improve any urinary problems. Women who have had babies will have been taught to tighten the muscles in the pelvic floor around the vagina. If you were not or you cannot remember how to do them, the practice nurse will have instruction leaflets. These exercises require discipline as they are boring and easy to forget. However, done regularly they can restore some bladder control and reduce the risk of leaking urine when sneezing or running.

Vaginal dryness

Vaginal dryness (see also Chapters 2 and 8) can become a problem for some women as they age. This can lead to pain on intercourse and a reluctance to have sex. This in turn can cause relationship problems and misunderstandings for some couples. Regular intercourse can help prevent vaginal dryness. When intercourse is painful, women tend to tense the muscles around the entrance to the vagina involuntarily, which further adds to the discomfort. Simple vaginal lubricants are available from pharmacies, and are very helpful. There is also a long-acting vaginal lubricant, also available from pharmacies, for women who need more continuous symptom relief. This has been shown to offer as much symptom relief as local vaginal oestrogen. (It is worth noting that very weak vaginal oestrogen preparations are available on prescription. These are absorbed only around the local area of the vagina and lower urinary tract without being absorbed generally in the body, so that they are safe for women who have a contraindication to systemic oestrogen. These vaginal oestrogen preparations can help the vaginal and urinary symptoms associated with the menopause.)

Other prescribed medication

In recent years it has been noticed that some medications that were developed or prescribed for other reasons can help reduce flushes and sweats. They include antidepressants and antiepileptics.

Antidepressants

Antidepressants such as paroxetine and venlafaxine have been shown to help alleviate symptoms of the menopause. They are usually prescribed in their smallest dose and benefits are usually felt within two weeks of starting them. However, as with any medication, there are side-effects, including dry mouth, nausea, constipation and reduced appetite. They can also offer a possible positive effect on mood and libido. Occasionally it may be appropriate to treat menopausal mood swings and insomnia with antidepressants or night sedation.

Antiepileptics

Gabapentin, an antiepileptic drug, is also useful in reducing hot flushes. More research on its effects is required. Other medications may be found to be helpful in due course, particularly when the cause of flushes is better understood.

Chapter 7
Staying healthy

Good health depends on many different things, and relates to the mind as well as to the body. While our physical health is mainly determined by the absence and prevention of disease, our mental health is dependent on many aspects of our lives: emotional, social, spiritual and intellectual. Numerous factors impact on our ability to stay healthy. In addition to the more obvious, such as diet and lifestyle, issues such as financial circumstances, social situation and outlook on life can also have an effect on our long-term well-being.

Life expectancy has increased dramatically in the Western world over the past hundred or so years. A woman's average life expectancy today is 83 years – so when she reaches the menopause at around the age of 50, she still has much of her life ahead of her. Unfortunately, health problems do increase with age, so it is very important to do everything possible to stay well, active and independent for as long as possible. Everyone needs to take some responsibility for his or her own health in this way.

In industrialised countries, by far the most common health problem in older people is heart disease (see Chapter 4 for more about this). Five times as many women die from heart disease, in particular coronary heart disease, as from breast cancer. It will kill one in every five women. Many people associate heart disease with the stereotype of the over-worked male executive, but in fact, after the menopause, heart disease becomes as common in women as it is in men. Furthermore, heart disease is more common among people doing boring repetitive jobs, who have no control over what they are expected to do, than in the high-powered, overworked executive. But, despite the high incidence of heart disease, there is much that we can do to help prevent it.

The other major health issue in women after the menopause is osteoporosis (see Chapter 3). Osteoporosis itself is not a cause of death; it is the fractures that occur as a result of the fragile bones that lead to so many other health and dependency problems. It is estimated that one in four women has osteoporosis by the age of 60 and half of all women have the condition by the age of 80. The bones that are most likely to fracture are the wrist, the vertebrae in the spine, and the hip. All fractures are painful.

Wrist fractures mean that sufferers generally need help with ordinary daily functions and chores for a few weeks until the injury has healed. Osteoporosis in the spine causes the vertebrae to become crushed. This in turn results in pain, loss of height and the stereotypical curved back or 'dowager's hump'. These changes are not reversible, and result in loss of mobility, reduced quality of life (but see Chapter 11 for details of new techniques such as kypho-plasty and vertebroplasty) and, for some, continuing pain. Hip fractures necessitate hospital admission, usually surgery, which carries risks in older people – as does the necessary immobility, because of the increased risk of deep vein thrombosis, large blood clots in the lung (pulmonary emboli, PE) and pneumonia. Most women never regain their former quality of life following a hip fracture.

These are sobering facts, but there are ways in which women can help to protect their health after the menopause, largely in terms of reassessing and adapting their diet and lifestyle. While it is true that changing what we eat and some of the ways in which we live requires discipline and commitment in the long term, diet and lifestyle are strongly implicated in disease and are part of the reason why cultures with different traditional diets and lifestyles have very different disease risks. An interesting study in the 1950s showed that Japanese immigrants to Hawaii who adopted the Hawaiian diet developed similar disease patterns to the native Hawaiians within one generation.

The weight issue

As the hormone levels change at the menopause, so does the body's shape. Women generally put on weight with age and particularly after the menopause, whether or not they take hormone replacement therapy (HRT). They tend to lose their 'hourglass' shape and become thicker around the waist and ribs. This change in fat distribution is associated with an increased risk of heart disease.

About one-third of British women, both pre- and post-menopausal, are overweight, and an additional 23 per cent are severely overweight or obese. Being overweight is a major risk factor for heart disease as it is linked with diabetes, high blood pressure and raised cholesterol levels in the blood. Other health issues associated with obesity are gall bladder diseases, osteoarthritis and other joint problems, breathing difficulties, urinary and gynaecological problems. Breast cancer is twice as common in post-menopausal women who are overweight. Other cancers associated with increased weight include cancers of the colon, endometrium (lining of the uterus) and gallbladder.

Osteoporosis, on the other hand, is more common in thin and petite women. These women might also be at greater risk of hip fracture following a fall because they have less fat protecting their hips. Having a weight within the normal range – neither too fat nor too thin – is the most healthy.

Many women find it harder to control their weight as they get older. The body's metabolism slows about 3 per cent with each decade, and so the calorie intake needs to be gradually decreased to compensate for this. Both diet and exercise are important for weight control, to ensure that more calories are not being consumed than are being used by the body for energy. In a recent study among overweight menopausal women who took up walking as exercise, the greatest weight loss was among those who exercised the most.

Body mass index

You can work out whether your weight is within a healthy range for you by using the body mass index (BMI) figures (see chart below). Although the BMI has some limitations, it provides a quick reference for the normal healthy weight range for a given height. In women who exercise regularly and have developed more muscle, however, it may show a misleading score. The acceptable range of body mass index – weight (kg), divided by height (m) squared – in women is between 20 and 23.5; in men it is between 20 and 25. A BMI of over 27 is associated with an increased risk of health problems such as high blood pressure, diabetes and heart disease. If this is the case, it would be wise to ask advice from a doctor about weight control.

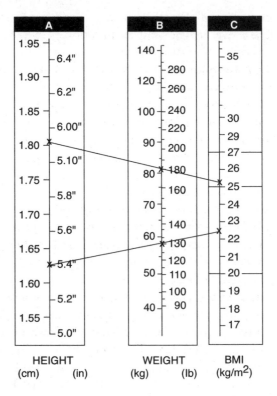

Figure 1   Body mass index

Diet

Food, for most people. is one of life's pleasures. However, the body's needs for specific nutrients changes with age, as it becomes less effective at absorbing some of the essential nutrients needed for health, and as the kidneys become less efficient at conservation. It is therefore increasingly important, as we get older, to eat some foods less frequently, particularly those that have a high fat and sugar content, and to eat more of others (e.g. fruit and vegetables).

Eating for a healthy heart

It has been known for a long time that diet is closely linked to heart disease. A varied diet with fresh fruits, vegetables and wholemeal products is likely to provide the daily requirements of vitamins and minerals that are significant for optimising cardiac health. At all stages of life it is wise to eat less fat and more fibre, and to reduce salt intake.

To **reduce fat intake**, avoid foods that are high in fat – such as cakes, pastry, biscuits and crisps. Grill or bake foods instead of frying them. If you have to fry food, then use a non-stick pan and use a vegetable oil, such as olive or sunflower. Always choose lean meat, poultry or fish. Eat poultry without its skin, which is where most of the fat is stored. Eat less saturated fat, which is present in fatty meats, chocolate and full-fat dairy products, as this type of fat is associated with high cholesterol levels, in particular higher levels of low density lipoproteins, which predispose to heart disease.

You can substitute these foods with skimmed or semi-skimmed dairy products and low-fat spreads that are high in polyunsaturated fat instead of butter.

It is recommended that everyone should eat at least five portions of fresh **fruit, vegetables or salad** daily. This does not include potatoes. The fruit and vegetables should be varied, as this is the best way to ensure that you receive all the important vitamins and minerals needed to provide heart protection.

Wholegrain carbohydrate foods such as wholegrain bread, pasta and rice provide both fibre and some of the essential B vitamins. These foods contain complex carbohydrates that take time for the body to digest and break down, so they tend to satisfy for longer and provide more constant and sustained blood-sugar levels.

Fibre is helpful to keep the bowels moving effectively, but excessive amounts of fibre may be associated with wind and prevent some nutrients being effectively absorbed, particularly calcium. One portion of oats (in porridge) or oatmeal daily has been shown to lower cholesterol. Potatoes are a valuable source of vitamin C particularly if the skins are eaten. However, you should avoid rich sauces, fillings and spreads with these carbohydrate foods.

High levels of **salt** can increase blood pressure, so avoid adding salt and using stock cubes or processed food. Try cooking without salt and flavour food with herbs and spices instead.

Research done since the mid-1980s has shown that **oily fish** eaten at least once a week is significant in reducing mortality from coronary heart disease. This is because fish is a rich source of mega-3 fatty acid, an unsaturated fat that is highly protective against heart disease. Inuit Indians, eating a traditional oily diet mainly consisting of fish, have a low incidence of heart disease.

Garlic preparations are a very popular over-the-counter product for reducing cholesterol. The scientific evidence, however, is unconvincing, although it is true that in Mediterranean countries, where people's diets do include a lot of garlic, there is a lower rate of heart disease than in the UK.

The vitamin debate

Vitamins and minerals are naturally occurring substances that are required in only very small amounts but which are essential for the normal, healthy functioning of the body. There are approximately 13 major vitamins and 25 essential minerals needed in the diet.

Vitamins are classified by simple alphabetical letters, although vitamin B is actually a group of vitamins rather than a single one. The main vitamins are A, the B group, C, D and E. Vitamin K is also important but it is formed by natural bacteria in the gut and is not eaten. The vitamins can be divided into two groups: the fat-soluble vitamins (A, D and E), which can be stored in the body; and water-soluble vitamins (B group and C), which, because they dissolve in water, cannot be stored by the body for so long. We all need a regular intake of vitamin C daily.

Minerals are inorganic substances that are found in the soil from which foods grow. Minerals too can be divided into two groups. There are those that the body needs in larger amounts, such as calcium and iron, and those that are only needed in small amounts, such as selenium. The latter are termed trace elements.

Lately there has been a huge increase in interest in vitamins and minerals within the medical profession and also among the general public. Dietary supplements containing multivitamins and minerals are being increasingly used in the belief that they improve general good health. As mentioned in Chapter 6, a study in 2002 indicated that 65 per cent of women over 60 years of age used food supplements but that two-thirds of this group did not associate the vitamin use with possible side-effects, which is slightly worrying. Vitamins and minerals are chemicals and as such have the potential for harm as well as good. Although the number of medical papers on the subject has mushroomed over recent years, there is still only limited knowledge on the benefits and safety of these supplements.

Vitamins and minerals are linked to health, including health of the heart. It is advisable to ensure an adequate intake of vitamins by eating a wide variety of the right amounts of fresh fruit and vegetables, carbohydrate and protein. Some research has shown that vitamins are important for the heart, particularly vitamins A, C and E (called the 'ACE vitamins'), in addition to some minerals such as selenium. By-products of the body's metabolism can produce substances called free radicals, which damage healthy cells, increasing the risk of heart disease and also some cancers. One large study in 1993 of nurses in the USA found that those who had taken vitamin E supplements for two or more years had 40 per cent lower rates of heart disease. In the same study, there was a more modest reduction in heart disease in nurses who had taken vitamin C. However, not all the evidence that the ACE vitamins can help reduce these health problems is consistent. In another heart study, vitamin supplements did not reduce the risk of heart disease or cancer, although they did not seem to have any harmful effects either.

It is debatable whether vitamin and mineral supplements should be recommended. One argument for supplementation is that it serves as a 'nutritional insurance'. Our bodies need adequate amounts of vitamins (particularly the ACE vitamins) and minerals to protect them from exposure to environmental pollutants and free radicals. However, it could be said that this can be done equally well by increasing the variety of fresh foods eaten.

Eating for strong bones

During childhood and adolescence the bones are growing in size, and bone mass continues to increase until a person reaches his or her thirties. But, as described in Chapter 3, because bones are living tissue they are being constantly renewed throughout a person's life. Although to some extent bone size and strength is determined by genetic factors, the long-term health of our bones is also influenced by diet and lifestyle.

It is therefore important to maintain an adequate **calcium** intake throughout adolescence, adulthood and into later years. (See the table in Chapter 3 for details of calcium-rich foods.) This is partic-ularly important for elderly people, for several reasons. As people get older, and particularly for women after the menopause, calcium is absorbed with more difficulty from the gut, so a higher calcium intake is needed to compensate. Also, the kidneys of older people become less efficient at saving calcium and so more is lost in the urine. A small amount of calcium is required constantly by the bloodstream for the effective functioning of muscles and nerves, and, in people of any age with inadequate levels of calcium, it may be removed from the bones if it is necessary in order to maintain this level in the blood.

Although a high calcium intake at and after the menopause cannot completely halt the bone loss at this time, it can slow it. Ultimately, this might make the difference, in old age, between having a fracture or not. An assessment of a number of studies has shown that a calcium intake of at least 1,000mg daily in menopausal women reduces the risk of hip fracture by 22 per cent.

At the time of writing, the recommended daily allowance of calcium for adults, as advised by the Department of Health, is 700mg. The British Menopause Society★ recommends that menopausal women who are not on hormone replacement therapy should include 1,500mg of calcium in their daily diet. Calcium is most effectively absorbed in the gut from dairy products, but many women will find it impossible to eat sufficient quantities of dairy products to maintain a daily intake of 1,500mg (the equivalent of two pints of milk), so a calcium supplement may be the only way to achieve this.

It has long been recognised that salt increases the risk of calcium loss by the kidneys. However, an average salt intake of 9g daily has been shown not to have any adverse effect on the bones. This level is in keeping with the low-salt diet that is recommended for a healthy heart. The National Osteoporosis Society (NOS)★ notes too that excessive quantities of caffeine or animal protein (i.e. meat or dairy products) can also inhibit the body's ability to absorb calcium. High phosphate intake has also been linked to increased urinary calcium loss. Phosphorus is present in fizzy drinks and is probably a more significant risk factor in younger people, if they are drinking canned drinks instead of milk.

Vitamin D is also important. In postmenopausal women, the addition of vitamin D with calcium is significant in reducing the risk of fracture. This may be partly because of vitamin D deficiency in older women, owing to a tendency to spend less time outside in sunlight. (The body makes vitamin D through the action of sunlight on the skin, and this is our main source of this vitamin.) Some doctors recommend adding a daily supplement of 800iu of vitamin D to the 1,500mg of calcium for older women. Alternatively, it is possible to buy food fortified with vitamin D. A supplemental source of vitamin D is particularly important in the winter in the UK.

Several other nutritional deficiencies, such as deficiency in **magnesium, other minerals, vitamins** or **trace elements**, have been linked with osteoporosis, but studies are very limited.

Studies have examined the effects of **phytoestrogens** (see Chapter 10) on bone, but the results of studies on genistein (one type of phytoestrogen) and a synthetic phytoestrogen called ipriflavone on maintaining bone mass are conflicting, and further data are awaited.

In postmenopausal women, **protein** in the diet is essential to maintain the microscopic structure of the bone. Small amounts need to be eaten regularly.

Exercise

Keeping fit and active is important for heart and bone health, and there are also numerous other health advantages. Women who are more active are likely to weigh less and consume less alcohol, and are less likely to smoke. They are also more likely to have diets that contain less saturated fat, more fibre and more fruit and vegetables. More active women have lower blood pressure, less risk of diabetes and lower cholesterol, which in turn reduces the heart disease risk. One study indicated that the level of physical activity associated with lower rates of coronary heart disease is easily within the ability of almost all women. Exercise can also reduce depression and improve insomnia, and generally contribute to a greater feeling of well-being. Physical activity can also help older women keep more mentally active.

However, for a wide variety of reasons, few women in the UK take regular exercise. They may be too tired, too busy or just not sporty. As a result, two-thirds of women are so unfit that they cannot keep up a normal walking pace up a gradual slope without having to stop. Over three-quarters of women over 65 years cannot even walk on the level for any distance.

Exercise does not have to take place in a gym or at a class, and nor does it have to mean sport. Exercise includes brisk walking, jogging, cycling or swimming (although this is not bone protective), and many more activities besides. It is important, however, that exercise is introduced gradually and that it is geared to the individual.

Exercising for a healthy heart

The most important aspect of exercise for a healthy heart is that it regular and energetic enough. For cardiac health, exercise needs to be brisk enough to raise the heart rate to about 120 beats per minute. Exercise should be started gradually and geared to a woman's age and fitness and then gradually increased as appropriate. It can be started gently, perhaps for ten minutes about three times each week, then gradually increased for longer periods, more frequently and more energetically. Start each exercise session with a few minutes of gentle warm-up, followed by more intense exercise that raises the heart rate, and finally some more gentle 'cool down' exercise at the end.

The effect of regular exercise means that the heart-rate gradually becomes slower, so the amount of work that the heart does is reduced. Exercise helps reduce blood pressure, as exercised muscle needs less blood flow, and it also protects against the formation of **atheroma** (fat plaques inside the arteries that are associated with heart disease). Exercise also reduces the risk of blood clots or thromboses, another health risk that increases with age.

Exercise and bone health

Exercise throughout life is important for healthy bones. In early life, exercise helps increase the density of bone, and later on it helps to conserve it. Regular, weight-bearing exercise is effective in slowing the gradual long-term bone loss that is related to ageing. However, in order to slow the rate of bone loss when this is most rapid, immediately after the menopause, the exercise would need to be frequent and high-impact; more, in fact, than most women could manage.

Exercise needs to be geared to an individual's physical ability. The safest exercise is walking – because it puts less strain on the knees and hips, and there is less risk of falling and sustaining a fracture. Optimum levels of exercise needed for bone health, to slow gradual bone loss, are not precisely known but are in the region of 20 to 30 minutes, three to five times a week. And the exercise will only protect bones for as long as it is continued. (See Chapter 3 for more about exercise and bone protection.)

Many working women find it hard to find time to fit in sufficient, regular exercise. Some women feel that they are 'on the go' all the time anyway. However, a study examining the effects of different exercises on bone density showed, interestingly, that high sporting activity and vigorous housework were related to a higher bone density, whereas exercise undertaken in the course of most people's work or normal daily life did not have a significant impact on their bones. So it would seem that finding time to fit in more exercise (or more vigorous housework!) is important. With a bit of imagination it's not too difficult to find opportunities to take exercise: for example, brisk walking to the next bus stop before getting on the bus, or walking up stairs whenever possible.

Protection against hip fractures

Hip fractures are an ever-increasing risk for women as they get older. Not only do the bones become more fragile, but women are more likely to fall because of poor eye sight, poor balance or generally reduced mobility. One simple and inexpensive protective measure against such fractures is hip protectors: specially designed underwear with padding over the hip area. Studies into their use have shown disappointing results, partly owing to the design of the protectors and the reluctance of women to wear them or carers to put them on. It is hoped that as designs improve the use of these protectors will increase.

Other lifestyle issues

Smoking and, if it is done to excess, drinking alcohol, exacerbate menopausal symptoms and compound the long-term health effects of the menopause.

However, changing one's drinking and smoking habits can be enormously difficult and not just because of the addiction factor. For some people, stopping one or other of these activities may be akin to removing one of life's greatest pleasures. It may also have a significant impact on one's social life. For these reasons, the support of friends and family is vital. It may be worth contacting your GP, practice nurse or smoking helpline for advice and support.

Smoking

About a quarter of British women smoke and more teenage girls than boys smoke. But smoking is a major contributor to heart disease and also to osteoporosis.

Smoking is responsible for 50 per cent of all avoidable deaths, half of these due to heart disease.

The nicotine in tobacco is thought to be toxic to the cells in bone that are responsible for the formation of new bone, and smokers are more likely to have lower bone mass than non-smokers. Smoking is also linked to an earlier menopause: smokers' periods finish one-and-a-half to three years earlier than non-smokers. This means that the bodily changes that take place at the menopause, such as bone loss, will start earlier.

Smoking also has an effect on oestrogen metabolism – the way that the body can use oestrogen. Smokers tend to have more hot flushes and sweats at the menopause, and for women taking hormone replacement therapy (HRT) in tablet form, smoking can reduce the effect of the medication.

Alcohol

Excessive alcohol, more than the recommended 14 units per week (one unit is equivalent to a glass of wine, a measure of spirits or half a pint of beer), is a well-known risk factor for osteoporosis. Alcohol has a toxic effect on the bone cells, as does smoking. Alcohol is also linked to malnutrition, as people who drink heavily may not have a balanced diet with sufficient essential nutrients. Alcohol can hinder the absorption of calcium from the gut and reduces the effectiveness of vitamin D.

Alcoholic drinks are high in calories, so weight gain is highly likely. Heavy drinking can also lead to diabetes. Excessive alcohol can trigger abnormal heart rhythms and very heavy drinking may actually cause heart failure because of its effect on heart muscle.

Alcohol is a diuretic and may increase urinary problems in some women, such as the urgent need to pass urine or having to get up at night to do so. As discussed in Chapter 6, alcohol makes hot flushes worse.

Caffeine

Recent research indicates that caffeine is not detrimental to bones, so long as the calcium content in the diet is adequate. However, caffeine is a stimulant and may contribute to insomnia. Caffeine has a diuretic effect and, like alcohol, can add to urinary problems.

Stress

Everyday life, for many women, is potentially stressful in many ways. Coping with a job and a home can be trying enough but there may be added pressures from the family, elderly parents and grand-children, as well as financial worries, relationship problems, bereavements and so on. Personality also plays a part: for example, some women are perfectionists, driving themselves very hard, or are sensitive or anxious. Others may be highly strung or have a confrontational personality, for example. Long-standing disap-pointments, regrets or disagreements can all play a part.

Stress can contribute to depression and anxiety problems. In isolation, stress is not a risk factor for heart disease but can contribute to it when combined with other factors such as high blood pressure, inactivity and being overweight.

Sometimes it is possible to limit the stress on oneself by making life changes, but often there is little that can be done in this way, at least in the short term. So the other way to approach stress is to try to limit its impact. Very simple methods such as making some time for yourself – for just a hot relaxing bath or a chat with a friend – or finding a hobby or interest, or taking up some form of exercise, can ease the pressure. Other options for managing stress include relaxation techniques or tapes, yoga or other complementary and alternative medicine (CAM) such as massage, aromatherapy, reflexology, acupuncture, shiatsu or t'ai chi (see also Chapter 6). There are many forms of CAM so it should be possible for any individual woman to find one that is right for her. Bear in mind that different therapies involve different amounts of physical contact with the practitioner, and it is important that you feel comfortable with the therapist. Consult your GP and make sure that the therapist keeps the GP informed of progress. When choosing a therapist, check that he or she is qualified and insured. Ask the therapist for his or her experience in treating people with similar problems to yours and ask how many sessions or how frequently you will need to be seen. Most of the major CAMs have a governing body that controls training and standards. For more information see *The Which? Guide to Complementary Therapies.*

If there are unresolved issues or problems that you know are affecting your mood and stress levels, it might be worth discussing these with your GP and considering dealing with them in other ways, such as by counselling.

Support networks

In many cultures, people commonly live in extended families, which provide the older generations with both social and practical support. This is much more unusual in the industrialised world. For this reason, getting older may, for some, mean the prospect of a lonely and isolated time. Also, alas, our society values youth over age, and does not offer the dignity and respect to older people that are apparent in some other parts of the world. But despite this, older people have so much to offer society in terms of experience, enthusiasm and time, and this is not unrecognised. A positive attitude is invaluable.

Whether or not it is possible to live close to family, it is well worth becoming involved in the local community and local events, which in turn will lead to activities, interests, friendships and purpose. Find out what is gong on through local libraries, sports centres, charities, community centres, religious institutions, local halls, local papers, councils or the Internet.

Sexual health

The menopause does not mean the end of an enjoyable and satisfying sex life. Sexuality is lifelong, and people of all ages have physical and emotional needs. Each couple is unique and the expression of their physical relationship will vary, but the way they fulfil their sexual needs may change with time – perhaps with a gradual decline in the frequency of intercourse, although the need for close physical contact may not diminish.

As discussed in Chapter 2, after the menopause, as a result of the lower oestrogen levels, the vagina tends to become drier and less elastic. For this reason intercourse may be less comfortable. However, regular sexual activity helps to keep the vagina more lubricated and elastic. If dryness is a problem then simple water-based vaginal lubricants are available from pharmacists. If you find that these are insufficient, speak to your GP or practice nurse; GPs can prescribe local oestrogen creams (see Chapter 5).

Sexually transmitted disease

The pattern of sexual relationships among older people in our society is changing dramatically. The rising divorce rate, with a third of marriages breaking up, means that people in their forties and fifties are now starting new relationships, with a much higher rate of sexual intercourse than previously. One disturbing consequence of this is that the age group with the fastest increase in the rate of sexually transmitted disease (STDs) in the UK at present is the over-50s. This is largely because the need for any contraception ceases two years after the menopause, so postmenopausal women are having unprotected sex. It is important that postmenopausal women still insist on condom use, for their own protection against STDs, unless there is no risk of acquiring a STD from their partner. See Chapter 8 for more on STDs.

Contraception

Women who are entering into new relationships in their forties or fifties may not have required contraception for the last decade or so – if, for example, their husband has had a vasectomy – so this may be an important time for reviewing contraceptive measures.

HRT is not a contraceptive. The advice from the Royal College of Obstetrics and Gynaecologists is that a woman should use contraception for two years after her menopause (remembering that the definition of menopause being no periods for a year) if she is below the age of 50, and that she should use contraception for one year after her menopause if she is over the age of 50. With the increasing number of women on the combined oral contraceptive pill, the 'mini' progestogen-only pill, and the intrauterine contraceptive system (IUCS), or on perimenopausal HRT with withdrawal bleed (see Chapter 5), it is sometimes very difficult to know when the menopause has actually occurred. If you are in any doubt, this should be discussed with your GP.

The following section outlines the options for contraception for perimenopausal and postmenopausal women.

Condoms

Condoms are a useful barrier method and also offer protection from infection with Human Immunodeficiency Virus (HIV), Human Papilloma wart Virus (HPV), and bacterial genial infections. However, if the vagina is very dry there is a high risk of ruptured condoms, and if this is the case lubricating spermicidal gels (see page 123) are recommended in combination with condoms. It should be remembered that some spermicides and vaginal lubricants (for example, baby oil), can cause condoms to split. Women can obtain free condoms from a family planning clinic but, owing to a quirk of the National Health Service, GPs cannot prescribe them.

Diaphragms or caps

Diaphragms are another good method of barrier contraception. They offer slight protection against STDs, but not as much as condoms. They require some skilled explanation on how to use them, which can be obtained from a GP or family planning clinic. They also require a certain degree of willingness to touch one's own genital area, which may be disagreeable to some women. If the vagina is very dry or there is a prolapse (see Chapter 8), a diaphragm might be technically difficult to fit. A possible side-effect of diaphragm use can be cystitis (urinary infection), but if so this implies that the diaphragm does not fit properly.

A diaphragm should be used in conjunction with a spermicide, and these are useful for vaginal lubrication. However, some spermicides can rot the rubber, leading to increased rupture of diaphragms or condoms, so it is important to check this with your family planning doctor or GP.

Diaphragms and spermicides can be obtained free of charge from your own GP or from a family planning clinic. The rubber does perish, so a new diaphragm is needed each year, no matter how little use it has had. This is also a useful check to make sure it still fits properly.

It is worth making a note of the size of the diaphragm – its diameter in millimetres – in your diary. This helps future reordering. The size is on the box, and in a little triangle on the diaphragm itself, but this can get obscured after much use. In an emergency, a diaphragm can be bought over the counter at a pharmacist, but it is essential to obtain the right size.

Spermicides

Spermicides are useful to assist vaginal lubrication. It is not sufficient to use them as a contraceptive method by themselves; they should be used with either condoms or diaphragms. Occasionally women get an allergic reaction to the spermicide: every time after use, the vagina becomes very sore and red. This can easily be mistaken for thrush. The solution is to either change the spermicide or to not use one. The active ingredients of the spermicide are listed on the tube and box, and a change to something different can help. The pharmacist should be able to advise on this.

Intrauterine devices (IUDs)

The intrauterine device, or 'coil' is usually made of plastic and/or copper. It is inserted into the uterus by a doctor, and should be checked yearly by a GP or family planning practitioner. If an intrauterine device is inserted after the age of 45, it may be safely left in until the menopause rather than being changed every three to five years as stated on the packet. This is because the risk of new infection being introduced by a new coil is greater than the risk of pregnancy with the old coil. Occasionally, coils cause heavy irregular bleeding and/or infection, and then they must be removed. Since intrauterine coils act by preventing the fertilised egg from implanting in the uterus, to some women they are ethically unacceptable. They also do not prevent conception in the Fallopian tube, so there is a risk of an ectopic pregnancy (where the egg implants in the Fallopian tube). They should not be used for women who have already had an ectopic pregnancy, as these women are at a higher risk of another. The failure rate for IUDs as a contraceptive in the perimenopausal age group is about 1 per cent.

Intrauterine contraceptive systems (IUCS)

This is a new sort of intrauterine system that has progestogen in the plastic core. It acts as a contraceptive and can 'switch off' the lining of the uterus, to produce very light periods or even no periods. It is therefore an invaluable treatment for perimenopausal women who have very heavy bleeding (see Chapter 8). It may be technically difficult to fit in women with fibroids (see Chapter 2) that project into the uterine cavity, or women who have not given birth (or who have done so by caesarean section), because it is very slightly wider than the usual IUD copper coils.

This method is a true contraceptive, in that it prevents conception, as opposed to ordinary coils, which prevent implantation of the egg, and so it may be more ethically acceptable to some women. There is also a very much lower risk of ectopic pregnancy, so these coils can be fitted in women who have already had an ectopic pregnancy. Since it gives a low dose of progestogen, some women experience breast tenderness, irregular menstrual spotting, and even acne. Some find that their premenstrual tension is worsened, although others find that it is eradicated by this method.

The IUCS is being used to provide the progestogenic part of hormone replacement therapy (see Chapter 5) in some women, although it has not received a licence for this yet.

Combined oral contraceptive pill

The low-dose combined oral contraceptive pill contains oestrogen and progestogen. It carries a small risk of stroke, heart attack and clots in the legs, which does increase in women with age and smoking. GPs may refuse to prescribe the oral contraceptive pill to older, smoking women, on the grounds that the risk is too great. For women who do not smoke and have no problems with their blood pressure or obesity, the combined oral contraceptive pill may be used until their mid-forties or even fifties. There may be a slight increased risk of breast cancer with continuous use, but recent studies have found no evidence for this. There may, however, be an increase in the risk of heart disease, strokes and deep vein thrombosis.

The progestogen-only 'mini' pill

The 'mini' pill is weaker than the combined pill as it contains only progestogen. In women in their forties and fifties it is as effective a contraceptive as the combined pill; providing, of course, that it is taken at the same time every day (within a three-hour window), with no missed pills. There is no upper age limit for use, and it can be used in women who have had a previous deep vein thrombosis.

Intramuscular 'depot' progestogens

This is an injection of progestogen that is given every three months, into the arm or bottom. Some women do not like depot injections as it causes them to feel bloated or have erratic periods. Other women prefer the simplicity of this method, and it also may stop heavy bleeding. In some women periods may stop completely; in others they may be light and irregular (and for some they are heavy and irregular). The disadvantage of stopping regular bleeds is that there is then uncertainty as to when the menopause has occurred.

Sterilisation

Sterilisation is now the most common form of contraception for couples in the UK in the perimenopausal age group. For men, vasectomy (cutting of the tubes that lead from the testicles to the penis) can be performed under a local anaesthetic. The man usually needs to take two or three days off work after the operation. A man is not infertile for about three months after sterilisation as there could still be some sperm swimming around in the tubes on the other side of the cut. The clinic that performs the sterilisation will require a sperm count after two or three months to check the absence of sperm from the ejaculate. The couple must use alternative contraception until a negative sperm count is achieved.

It is surprising how often women forget that if, their partner is sterilised, this does not mean that they (the women) are infertile, and that they must use contraception if having sex with someone else.

For women, sterilisation involves the tying or clipping of the Fallopian tubes. This is done with a laparoscope (a small telescope) inserted through a tiny hole into the abdomen by the navel. This can be done providing there is no previous surgery in the abdomen that could have caused scars or adhesions internally, which are difficult to get past. A previous Caesarean section, for example, or other gynaecological or bowel or bladder surgery, may make this procedure technically much more difficult – as does extreme obesity.

Women who are sterilised should use contraception up the point of sterilisation. This is to avoid the theoretical risk of an egg going into the uterus after the fallopian tubes have been tied.

There is a small failure rate with either female (0.03 per cent) or male sterilisation. Either is difficult to reverse, so this must be assumed to be an irrevocable change.

Natural family planning
Although women with a lot of commitment can use natural family planning reliably in their thirties, it is not appropriate during the perimenopause. This is because natural family planning relies on a predictable menstrual cycle. In the transition of the perimenopause to the menopause, women's hormones are in chaos and their cycles become unpredictable. Methods relying on the detection of hormonal changes at ovulation are therefore very unreliable and cannot be recommended. Temperature changes are inconsistent, and women who have previously been able to judge ovulation by their vaginal mucus changes also find that these cease to be typical.

Chapter 8

Increased health risks at the menopause

The menopause brings increased risk not only of osteoporosis (see Chapter 3) and cardiovascular disease (see Chapter 4), but also of irregular periods, endometriosis, ovarian disease, urinary infections, diabetes and thyroid disorders among others. However, the majority of women will experience few, if any, of these conditions.

Irregular periods and bleeding

As pointed out in Chapter 2, women approaching the menopause often experience irregular periods. While this is normal, irregular bleeding is not. Any bleeding between periods, after the menopause or after intercourse should be discussed with a doctor.

Women under the age of 54

Erratic periods

Between the ages of 46 and 54 it is common to have irregular periods. You could, say, have a period, then no bleeding for three months, followed by two heavy bleeds in six weeks and then nothing again for another four months. This is the result of the natural process of the menstrual system winding down.

Amenorrhoea

Amenorrhoea (or the absence of periods) is, of course, the main sign of the menopause, and is to be expected sometime before the age of 55. Other reasons for this condition include extreme weight loss, a hyperactive thyroid and stress (see Chapter 1 for a list).

Painful periods

Painful periods, called dysmenorrhoea, are caused by severe cramping of the muscle wall of the uterus as it expels its lining, the endometrium.

Prostaglandins (hormone-like substances produced from fatty acids) are present in most body cells. They are identified, like vitamins, by a numbered letter. Prostaglandins alter body chemistry and their influence is widespread: they affect such areas as the heart, intestine, blood vessels and uterus. It is known that prostaglandins of the $F_{2\alpha}$ and E_2 series are responsible for menstrual cramps. Anti-prostaglandin drugs have been developed to reduce their effects. Examples are mefenamic acid (Ponstan) and naproxen sodium (Synflex). These medications can ease troublesome menstrual cramps.

Abdominal pain that occurs when there is no period is likely to be caused by fibroids, endometriosis, ovarian disease or pelvic or urinary infection (see sections on these conditions below for details).

Heavy periods

If your periods are extremely heavy and you are not taking hormone replacement therapy (HRT), go and see your GP. You might be anaemic (see 'Anaemia' on page 147), or have a polyp (see 'Cervical erosions and polyps', on page 139) and might need treatment to lessen the flow.

If you have been taking HRT for at least four months and your periods are intolerably heavy, your GP could try giving you another preparation with a different progestogen which might suit you better. If you still require contraception, the levonorgestrel-releasing intrauterine device may be a reasonable solution because it has the added advantage of stopping periods.

Drug treatments for heavy periods

- **Non-steroidal anti-inflammatory drugs (NSAIDs)**
  A systematic review (12 randomised controlled trials involving 313 women) showed that these drugs – all members of the aspirin family, e.g. mefenamic acid (Ponstan), ibuprofen (Neurofen) – reduced blood loss. NSAIDs have the additional benefit of relieving period pain too. They suit women who do

not want to take hormones and who wish to take something only during a period, not continuously. Some NSAIDs are sold over the counter and so women have immediate access to treatment. In randomised controlled trials, 50 per cent of women taking NSAIDs experienced indigestion, nausea, vomiting and/or diarrhoea, but similar levels were found in those taking a placebo. Some people are allergic to NSAIDs and those who have asthma may find that their condition is aggravated by these drugs.

- **Tranexamic acid** This is another treatment that has been shown to reduce heavy periods. Tranexamic acid is not a hormone, and is only taken during heavy menstruation. However, unlike NSAIDs, it does not help period pain but only blood loss. A third of those treated in trials reported nausea or leg cramps.

- **Levonorgestrel intrauterine contraceptive system (IUCS)** The levonorgestrel IUCS reduces menstrual blood loss by 80–90 per cent after about six months of use. In one randomised controlled trial involving 56 women, 64 per cent of those on a waiting list for hysterectomy cancelled their surgery after being fitted with a levonorgestrel IUCS compared with 14.7 per cent in the control group. A drawback is that it needs to be fitted, which can be uncomfortable and carries a small risk of perforation of the uterus. It is technically difficult to introduce an IUCS into a uterus that has not experienced a vaginal delivery (as the cervix is smaller), or one that has large fibroids (as the uterine cavity can be distorted). A levonorgestrel-releasing IUCS can produce irregular, continuous bleeding for the first six months. The side-effects are progestogenic, that is, you might experience irregular spotting, tender breasts, increased premenstrual tension, acne, weight gain and increased mood swings. It is a licensed form of contraception (see Chapter 7).

For women over 55: postmenopausal bleeding

If you have not had any periods for a year, and then have a period, or even just some spotting or a yellowy discharge, you should get this checked by your GP. Irregular bleeding after the menopause (postmenopausal bleeding) is always taken seriously as there is a very tiny risk that it could be an early sign of endometrial cancer

(cancer of the uterus or womb). For every 100 women that experience abnormal bleeding around menopause, 90 will have completely benign causes for this (a dry, sore vagina or a polyp, see below). The women who do have abnormal cells in the uterus can usually be fully cured by surgery. Risk factors for endometrial cancer are not having any children, obesity, and early age of first having periods.

Your GP should do an internal examination and look at the neck of the uterus with a speculum, like when you have a cervical smear, to see if there are any polyps. He or she may either refer you to a gynaecological clinic or arrange an outpatient ultrasound to check the thickness of the lining of the uterus, and possibly a biopsy (see Chapter 9).

Conditions of the uterus and the ovaries

Endometriosis

When the endometrium (the lining of the uterus) is shed each month, most of the cells drop through the vagina, and out of the body. This is a period. However, a few trickle back from the uterus down the Fallopian tubes and find their way into the abdominal cavity. These little cells grow there forming small cysts on the inside abdominal wall, the bowel and the bladder, and in the space between the vagina and the back passage (rectum) called the Pouch of Douglas. This process is known as endometriosis. These little pockets of growing cells take on a monthly cycle like the rest of the lining of the uterus so that women quite often feel bloated or experience abdominal pain a few days before a period in the same place each month (often low back or between the legs), and may notice occasional black tar-like vaginal discharge. This is one of the endometrial cysts bursting, and discharging through the vagina.

Almost all women have some endometriosis in the abdominal cavity. It can almost be seen as a consequence of having periods. What is less clear is why an unlucky small percentage have severe abdominal pain with endometriosis, and other women do not. It may relate to where the patches of endometriosis are in the body. Endometriosis usually starts when a woman is in her late 20s. During the menopause these pockets of endometriosis shrivel up, so ceasing to be a problem, unless you choose to prolong the hormonal stimulation by taking HRT. The National Endometriosis Society* is an active self-help group.

Fibroids

Fibroids are thickened bulges of the muscular wall of the uterus (the myometrium) which cause a bump or protrusion. They can be on the outside of the uterus, in the uterine wall or projecting into the internal cavity of the uterus. Most women over the age of 40 have fibroids, which are completely benign and usually symptomless. Very large fibroids can press on the bladder, causing urinary symptoms, or can push the uterus down though the pelvic floor, leading to a prolapse (see below). Sometimes the fibroids prevent the walls of the uterus contracting efficiently during a period, leading to heavier periods, which in turn can cause anaemia and therefore tiredness. In such cases, a hysterectomy might be considered to be the best solution.

Hysterectomy

A hysterectomy is the surgical removal of the uterus. As its name suggests, a total hysterectomy is removal of the whole uterus. A subtotal hysterectomy is one in which the cervix (the neck of the uterus) is left behind. A hysterectomy can be performed from an incision in the low abdomen, along a line where 'brief' knickers would be. The uterus can also be removed in some women through the vagina (thus avoiding an abdominal scar) with a laparoscope. The death rate for a hysterectomy is 1 in 2,000 in women under 50 years who have a hysterectomy for non-malignant conditions. Major or minor adverse effects are reported in a third of women: generalised infection (sepsis), urinary tract infections, urinary retention, requirement for blood transfusion, collections of blood around the wound (haematoma), post-operative pain, and an earlier menopause even if the ovaries are conserved, owing to post-operative ovarian failure.

131

Benign ovarian disease

The ovaries are active organs that produce an egg each month by ripening a cyst, which bursts to release the ovum. Ovarian cysts are quite common and are usually found when an ultrasound investigation is being performed. Benign ovarian cysts can vary in size, from holding 1 cubic centimetre of fluid to several litres. They can twist or rupture, causing agonising acute abdominal pain, but this is very rare. Usually a skilled ultrasound technician can tell by ultrasound alone the difference between a completely benign fluid-filled cyst and a malignant one. If there are any doubts then a laparoscopy and biopsy are performed.

After the menopause ovarian activity dies down, so it is much less common to find hormonally driven ovarian cysts. Usually all cysts present after the menopause are investigated to exclude ovarian cancer.

Prolapse of the uterus

The supporting ligaments of the uterus and vagina, which may have been stretched by childbirth, become weaker as the menopause approaches. The dwindling supply of oestrogen in the menopausal years also reduces the elasticity and firmness of tissue and skin, allowing the uterus to descend into the mid- and lower vagina. Varying degrees of prolapse are thus produced. A loose pouch of vaginal skin, like an inverted pocket, with the bladder attached, may protrude into the cavity of the vagina: this is a cystocele. A similar prolapse of the bowel and back wall of the vagina is called a rectocele. Either condition, if severe, may require corrective surgery, in the form of an anterior or posterior repair.

Urinary disorders

As pointed out in Chapter 2, infections of the urinary tract may occur at any time of life, but because the lining walls of these areas tend to become thin at the menopause, susceptibility to infection is increased. Moreover, urinary incontinence (see also Chapter 9) could become a problem as women grow older.

Pelvic floor laxity

One can explain the problems of a lax pelvic floor as a failure of evolution to cope with humans standing upright. In mammals that stand on four legs gravity usually keeps the abdominal organs slung in the abdomen. Standing upright means that all the pressure of the abdomen is put on the weak muscles of the pelvic floor. Over time the muscles get laxer, thinner and weaker, which causes the whole pelvis floor to sag and loosen. This is rather like the webbing in a favourite old arm chair that sags after many years of use. Structures such as the bladder or uterus which are supposed to be supported sitting on the pelvic floor can therefore fall through it.

Oestrogen has a marked effect on collagen throughout the body, which is why face texture gets more wrinkly after the menopause with lower oestrogen levels. Collagen provides the ropes that tie all the organs together and keep them mobile but fixed. Interestingly, collagen varies across families and some people have a genetically different collagen to others. It is therefore useful to ask older female relatives in the family whether they have suffered from pelvic floor problems. Another factor in a drooping pelvic floor is childbirth and the size of the baby. Carrying around an extremely large baby in the uterus bouncing on to the pelvic floor is not good for the

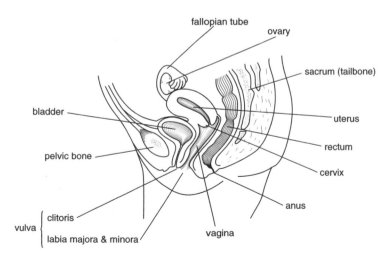

Figure 1 Female reproductive system

muscles. Women are taught pelvic floor exercises postnatally but few have the time to do them. Often, women experience their first urinary incontinence during pregnancy and after childbirth. In fact, childbirth significantly damages the pelvic floor muscles and can even damage the muscles that keep the bladder and the back passage continent (i.e. not leaking). If a woman goes to her GP with urinary or faecal incontinence she will be asked about how many pregnancies she has had, how heavy the babies were and what the mode of delivery was. For details of examinations conducted by the doctor see Chapter 9.

Treatment options

- **Pelvic floor exercises** These exercises, also known as Kegel's exercises after the physician who devised them, involve learning to squeeze the pelvic floor muscles for increasing lengths of time to tone up the muscles and improve bladder control. Pregnant women are usually taught these exercises as part of the antenatal classes they attend. The technique is similar to stopping yourself in the middle of passing urine and holding the stream before letting go again. If you are experiencing stress incontinence, you need to do these exercises for three to six months before you notice any improvement, and should continue to do them indefinitely. If you have not been taught these exercises, ask at your surgery if there is a continence clinic that has specialist physiotherapists.
- **Vaginal ring pessary** For women who have slight pelvic floor laxity a plastic polymer ring can be inserted into the upper vagina to buttress the bladder and uterus. The ring needs to be changed by your GP every six months. Unfortunately, some women have such a lax vagina that they cannot retain a ring. In such cases surgical intervention may need to be considered. The ring does not get in the way of sexual intercourse and, once inserted, should be completely comfortable and painless.
- **Surgery** Various surgical techniques are available to help women with incontinence problems. One of the newest is one in which a tape is threaded around the bladder to hoist it back up into the pelvis. It is the least invasive surgery, and is suitable even for women over 90. The surgeon should discuss all the

options with you, including hysterectomy and bladder repair. You need to know the success rates for the operation for a five-year period: these vary between surgeons, centres and type of surgery.

Cystitis

Cystitis, a urinary tract infection, is most commonly caused by a bacteria called E.coli, which is present in everyone's bowel. It is very much more common in women than men, because the urethra (the tube through which the urine passes from the bladder to the opening in the vagina) is much shorter in women and so bacteria are much more likely to creep up into the bladder from the outside world. The symptoms of cystitis are pain or burning on passing urine and a strong and frequent urge to urinate. The urine itself is often smelly and may be pink or even red with blood. Medical evidence shows that 50 per cent of cases of cystitis actually get better within 24 hours on their own because the body can fight the bacteria, but you should seek help immediately if you are pregnant or diabetic, or you know you have an abnormality of your kidney or your urinary system, or if you have a kidney stone. You should seek help within 24 hours if the symptoms of cystitis do not get better. The cure for cystitis is a short course of antibiotics. If you are not better within a day of taking the antibiotics it may be that that particular drug is not the right one for the organism and you need to go back to your doctor again.

The best way to avoid cystitis is to drink plenty of water (at least two litres) every day. Research has shown that even a small amount of cranberry juice taken last thing before going to bed can help reduce the rate of chronic urinary infections. This is because cranberry juice has a chemical in it that actually stops the bacteria sticking on to the inside of your bladder wall, so you can flush out the organisms more easily. Some women find they get more cystitis after sex, but this can be reduced if both partners wash before having sex and if the women gets up and urinates after sex, to flush out her bladder. If the occurrence of cystitis is very clearly sex-related, GPs sometimes give women antibiotics; taking just one dose after sex will stop an attack. Women who have recurrent urinary tract infections (i.e., more than three a year) need to have an ultrasound scan of the urinary system to check that there is no abnormality and then the possibility of a three-month course of low-dose antibiotics to try and get rid of the bacteria from the system.

Postmenopausal cystitis is quite common because the lack of oestrogen makes the urethra widen, thus encouraging bacteria to slide down it. Randomised controlled trials have shown that recurrent urinary tract infections in older women can be reduced by treatment with local oestrogen pessaries.

Urethral syndrome

It is not unusual for urinary and vaginal infections to be present together. It is possible that cross-infection between the vagina and the urinary tract is one cause of urethral syndrome. The definition of urethral syndrome is pain when passing water and greater frequency of urination, but with no bacteria found in the urine. In postmenopausal women the urethra can become extremely sore from a lack of oestrogen, and this can be successfully treated with local oestrogens (creams or pessaries) placed in the vaginal opening.

Vaginal discharge

The vagina normally produces fluid to keep it moist, and it has a natural acidity produced by special bacteria that live there. This acidity keeps infections at bay. If the bacteria are destroyed, by antibiotics or vaginal deodorants, or douching for example, or if the acidity is disturbed by pregnancy, the contraceptive pill or after the menopause, then vaginal infections become more likely.

Vaginal discharge may be normal (see below) or it may be caused by an infection. Medical help is available from your GP or from clinics (known as genito-urinary medicine clinics) that specialise in sexually transmitted diseases. GUM clinics are usually found in local hospitals and most offer a walk-in service, without the need for a letter from your GP. Staff will not communicate with your GP without your permission.

Normal discharge

Many women notice an increase in their normal discharge when they are pregnant, on the pill, at ovulation (two weeks before a period) or after intercourse. This is normal, and does not require any special treatment. Excessive washing may cause infections because it may destroy the normal bacteria and predispose you to thrush. Normal discharge does not smell, itch or cause any irritation to the vagina.

Main causes of vaginal discharge

Infective

- bacterial vaginosis
- Candida (thrush)
- chlamydia
- gonorrhoea
- trichomonas

Non-infective

- cervical ectropion (erosion)
- cervical polyp
- lost tampon
- miscarriage
- tumours of the cervix or uterus

Infective causes: causes and treatments

Cause	Type of discharge	Smell	Other symptoms
Thrush (Candida)	Creamy white	None	Itchy, sore vagina
Bacterial vaginosis	Grey-white and watery	Fishy – especially after sex	Vagina not sore
Trichomonas	Frothy and green	Foul-smelling	Sore vagina
Chlamydia	May not be any; may be thick and bloody	No smell usually	Fever, pain during intercourse, partner may have pain passing water
Gonorrhoea	May not be any; may be thick and bloody	Smelly	As chlamydia

Thrush

It is estimated that 75 per cent of women experience thrush at least once in their lifetime. The infection is caused by a yeast (Candida). It is more likely to occur if your immune system is low, after a course of antibiotics, if you are diabetic or pregnant, or if you have used some very alkaline bubble baths/scented soaps. Vulval itching and a thick white discharge which does not smell are the principal symptoms.

There are a number of antifungal agents which can be had on prescription or over the counter. If you have recurrent thrush (i.e., four episodes or more in one year), you should see your doctor to check that you have not become diabetic, and that your immune system is still working efficiently.

Bacterial vaginosis (BV)

This is the most common cause of a smelly vaginal discharge in women aged between 20 and 50. BV results from an exuberant overgrowth of bacteria which are normally present in small numbers. It is not a sexually transmitted disease, and is more common in smokers, and women who use vaginal douching and intrauterine devices. The most effective treatment is with metronidazole, an antibiotic which will make you exceedingly sick if you drink alcohol with it.

Trichomonas

This is a sexually transmitted infection, with low rates in the UK. A smelly discharge is the sign that makes women seek a medical consultation. Diagnosis can be made by taking a swab for culture. Treatment is with metronidazole. Partners must be treated too.

Chlamydia

Chlamydia is a sexually transmitted bacterial infection. It is most common in girls under 25 years. Diagnosis can be made by taking a swab from the cervix. Treatment is with antibiotics (doxycycline or azithromycin), and partners must be traced and treated too.

Gonorrhoea

Gonorrhoea is rarer than it was in the 1970s, but is making a comeback in girls aged 15–19. Diagnosis is by swab culture. Treatment is with antibiotics (ciprofloxacin, ofloxacin and ampicillin).

Non-infective causes

Cervical erosions and polyps

The cervix looks like a ring doughnut, the central hole being the entrance to the uterus. It is very common for a few cells from the lining of the uterus to creep out to live at the cervical opening. This makes the cervix look red, and produces a copious mucus discharge. This phenomenon is known as a cervical erosion or ectropion. Normally it does not require any treatment, as it is virtually a normal variant. However, if the vaginal discharge is very distressing, the cervix can be burnt with hot cautery, which stimulates regrowth of the cervical lining cells, thus reducing the erosion.

A polyp is a benign outgrowth of cells. Cervical polyps can cause bleeding on sexual intercourse and an increased vaginal discharge. They are usually on a slender stalk and can be simply twisted off by your GP, or gynaecologist in a clinic, without any anaesthetic.

Lost tampons

Women occasionally forget to remove a tampon when inserting a new one. So after a period has ended, a tampon is left behind, causing a very malodorous discharge. If you suspect that you might have a tampon left inside, go to your surgery: your GP will be able to see it easily using a speculum, and can remove it painlessly with a pair of long-handled sponge forceps.

Tumours

Tumours of the cervix or uterus are rare. However, they often cause a thin, yellow blood-flecked continuous discharge. Do not ignore such a sign. If detected early such tumours can be cured. Sometimes patients are too embarrassed to seek help and leave it a long time before seeking advice, which makes it harder to cure the condition.

Concerns about the breast

Most women fear breast cancer more than any other disease. We all have friends or relatives who have had breast cancer, as it is extremely common. One in nine women in the UK will have breast cancer at some point in their lives. Breast awareness, being aware of your breasts, how they change through a cycle and how they normally feel, has been a central feature of the government's efforts to help women see their doctors as soon as they detect a problem with their breasts (see Chapter 9). The national screening programme for breast cancer between the ages of 50 and 64 has also had a recent significant impact on lowering the death rate from breast cancer.

The normal breast

The breast changes in a monthly cycle in a premenopausal woman. In response to the oestrogen and progesterone secreted in the monthly cycle, towards the end of the cycle the breasts become heavy, slightly enlarged, more lumpy and noticeably tender. Often women can develop cysts (fluid-filled sacs) in the second half of the cycle. The sacs may be soft or firm depending on the tension of the fluid in the sac. They may be painful if they have developed rapidly, like a balloon under pressure. Usually cysts reduce in size after the period. Cysts can be aspirated by a general practitioner or a specialist breast clinic and the fluid sent for microscopic examination (see Chapter 9).

There is evidence that oil of evening primrose helps significantly with painful tender breasts (mastalgia). This can be bought over the counter in reputable chemists and health food shops.

Breast cancer

Some women have a very strong family history of ovarian and/or breast cancer. There is also a genetic link with bowel cancer in some families. These cancers tend to occur in younger women (those in their 30s and 40s). The vast majority of breast cancers occur after the menopause, and do **not** have a genetic cause.

Risk factors for breast cancer in women

The following factors are considered to increase the risk of breast cancer:

- family history of breast cancer
- obesity (a BMI of 30 doubles the risk of breast cancer)
- late menopause
- HRT use after the menopause

- not having children
- children born after the age of 35
- not having breastfed.

An important fact that is completely overlooked in the UK is that being fat doubles the risk of breast cancer. Obesity also increases a woman's risk of uterine cancer after the menopause. The reason for this increased risk is that fat women have much more fat (adipose) tissue which actually makes oestrogen, so measurable circulating levels of oestrogen are higher in fat women than in very thin women after the menopause. As both breast cancer and uterine cancer are hormonally driven, having a higher level of oestrogen makes the woman more likely to get the disease.

Women who have breast cancer

Most women in the UK who have breast cancer are given five years' treatment with tamoxifen if the tumour is 'oestrogen receptor positive'. Samples from the tumour are sent to the laboratory to see if it is hormonally driven. Some cancers are not hormonally driven and are insensitive to hormone receptor blockers. Many breast cancers are very sensitive to oestrogen and tamoxifen acts to block these oestrogen receptors, thus shrivelling up the cancer cells. Tamoxifen has had a remarkable impact on breast cancer survival in the Western world since its launch in the 1960s. It was the original oestrogen receptor modulator (SERM) and has now caused enormous interest in research for a perfect designer HRT that will both protect the breast against breast cancer as well as improve bone density and make women feel good (see Chapter 10). Tamoxifen improves bone density and so women who have had breast cancer and are on tamoxifen are protected from osteoporosis. Tamoxifen can slightly increase the risk of endometrial cancer, so if a women is taking tamoxifen and experiences irregular vaginal bleeding, she should be referred for tests on the endometrium.

The effect of the menopause on other cancers

With the success of modern medicine, many women survive cancer and then want to know whether they can take HRT or not, or how the menopause will affect them. The worrying issue of whether HRT causes different cancers is dealt with in Chapter 5. The sections below briefly describe some of the more common cancers and address the question of whether HRT might cause a recurrence of a cancer or cause a separate new cancer to develop.

A cancer 'recurs' because not every single malignant cell was removed or killed by the original treatments, which may have included surgery and/or radiotherapy and chemotherapy. Giving HRT cannot cause 'a recurrence' because the malignant cells are already there in the body, growing. However it may stimulate these malignant cells to grow faster. It is therefore medical advice **not** to give HRT if a person has an oestrogen-sensitive gynaecological tumour.

Endometrial cancer

Abnormal vaginal bleeding, especially after the menopause, can be a sign of cancer of the endometrium (womb lining). This is rare in women under 50, and is less common in women who have taken the contraceptive pill. It is more common in women who are childless, older than 50, obese or who have had a late menopause.

There is no evidence that the rare sarcomas of the uterus are oestrogen-sensitive.

It has been known since the 1960s that giving oestrogen alone to women who have a uterus can cause a higher rate of endometrial cancer. This is why women with a uterus need both oestrogen and progestogen. The progestogen protects the lining of the uterus. Indeed, sometimes women are treated with progestogens if they have an endometrial cancer.

If you have had a hysterectomy following endometrial cancer it is safe to take HRT afterwards, if you wish. Discuss the issues with your hospital specialist.

Cervical cancer

Abnormal vaginal bleeding may be a sign of cancer of the cervix. It is thought to be more common among women who have the wart virus (although not necessarily warts), those who start to have sex at an early age, and those who smoke. Having regular (minimum three-yearly) smear tests from the age of 20 helps to identify early changes that may eventually lead to cancer unless they are treated. Having a smear, waiting for the result and then being told that the result is abnormal can be very stressful, but the overall aim is to prevent cancer, so the stress is worth putting up with. Smears may be reported as 'inadequate', which means that the person taking the smear did not manage to get enough cells on the slide to allow a proper report. If that happens, you will be invited to have another smear. Having a smear when you are in mid-cycle helps to ensure that the smear is adequate. Smears may be reported as showing 'inflammation or severe inflammatory changes' which may mean an infection is present. Smears may show 'dyskaryosis', which can be mild, moderate or severe. These changes may never develop into cancer if they are left untreated, but there is a small chance that they will progress to localised cancer (carcinoma in situ) or to more extensive cancer. Because of this, treatment – usually laser treatment of the abnormal area – is advised if the abnormality is confirmed after further examination with a colposcope. A colposcope is a piece of equipment that allows the gynaecologist to look at a magnified view of the cervix.

Cancer of the cervix is an increasingly common condition in the UK. Up to one in ten women has had laser treatment on her cervix at some time in the past for early cell changes in the cervix. There is no evidence that women who have been treated for cervical cancer should not have HRT, particularly if they are prematurely menopausal from their treatment.

Ovarian cancer

Ovarian cancer does not usually cause abnormal vaginal bleeding. This type of cancer is difficult to detect because it does not cause many specific symptoms until it is well advanced and difficult to treat. Once it starts to spread to other organs it can cause abdominal pains, bloating, nausea, vomiting, pain on intercourse, erratic vaginal bleeding and bowel disturbances including diarrhoea, constipation or blockage of the bowel. It affects 5,000 women a year in the UK, and causes 4,000 deaths a year. It is more common among women who have a sister, mother or daughter who has had ovarian cancer or breast cancer which developed at a young age. Ovarian cancer is also more common among women who have never had children. It is less common among women who have been on the oral contraceptive pill and rare in women under 50; it becomes more common as women get older. The diagnosis is often made by chance if a woman has a vaginal examination or an ultrasound scan. Most ovarian cysts are totally benign and harmless. They may need to be removed in an operation to be certain that they are not cancerous. There is no specific screening test for ovarian cancer which is reliable, but women who have a family history of the disease should see a specialist who can advise about blood tests and regular ultrasound scans, which may help to pick it up at an early stage.

The treatment of ovarian cancer involves surgery to remove the growth, and further surgery to remove the womb, ovaries and tubes if the growth is cancerous. Chemotherapy, using powerful cancer-killing drugs, is also given.

Colorectal (bowel) cancer

Several studies have shown a decreased risk of bowel cancer in women taking HRT. This may be explained in terms of oestrogen receptors in the bowel; it has also been argued that the sort of women who take HRT are generally those who are very interested in their health and may have higher fibre, healthier diets than women who do not take HRT. More medical trials in the future will make this clearer, but certainly on the basis of available evidence there is no reason why women who have got bowel cancer should not take HRT.

Leukaemias and lymphomas

Some children and young women get leukaemia or lymphomas for which they have had chemotherapy and/or radiotherapy. This treatment may cause the ovaries to fail early. So even though such women may survive into adulthood, they might find themselves having a menopause at the age of 20. These women should be offered HRT until the age at which they would have had a natural menopause.

There are, of course, other issues involved, such as fertility. Research is being done at present to freeze wedges of ovary prior to cancer treatment, in the hope that the eggs can be used in the future (see Chapter 11).

The thyroid

The thyroid gland is the same shape and size, and sits in the same position, as a man's bow tie. It is controlled by a hormone produced by the brain called TSH (thyroid-stimulating hormone) which 'instructs' the thyroid gland to produce thyroid hormones. The thyroid hormones (thyroxine) circulate in the bloodstream and are responsible for driving many of the body's functions. Women are more prone to having too much or too little thyroid hormone than men for reasons which are not well understood but are linked to the presence of the female sex hormones.

Disorders of the thyroid

Thyroid disorders are often sparked off by hormonal crises, such as pregnancy and the menopause. It is more common to have an overactive thyroid (thyrotoxicosis) when young, and for it to 'burn out' into an underactive thyroid (myxoedema) when older, but sometimes even very old people can have an overactive thyroid.

Having an underactive thyroid is a little like having your car engine tuned too low; your whole body operates below par. This may result in weight gain, lethargy, shortness of breath, puffy ankles, feeling cold the whole time, thin hair, and heavy periods. A blood test confirms the diagnosis and treatment is by taking daily tablets to replace the thyroxine. Treatment needs to continue for life. Women normally feel very much better once their thyroid hormone levels return to normal.

Having an overactive thyroid is like having your car engine too highly tuned: your whole body is in overdrive. This may result in weight loss, shaking hands, sweatiness, palpitations, irritability and infrequent periods. In some forms of this condition, the eyes can look very bulging and staring. A blood test confirms the problem and further tests may be needed to see why the thyroid is overactive.

Investigations and treatment

After a blood test confirms what is wrong with the thyroid, treatment initially involves drugs to lower the thyroid hormones (carbimazole) and drugs to control the symptoms (such as propranolol for palpitations). Younger women may be offered an operation to remove part of the thyroid gland. This leaves a thin scar around the neck which can usually be easily covered by a necklace. Older women may be offered treatment with injections of radioactive iodine, which is absorbed by the thyroid gland and destroys some of the thyroid. Both forms of treatment may be so effective that a woman ends up with too little thyroid hormone and needs to take supplements of thyroxine to get the level right.

Maturity onset diabetes mellitus

Diabetes is also known as diabetes mellitus or 'sugar diabetes'. It is caused by a failure of the pancreas to produce sufficient insulin, the hormone responsible for breaking down carbohydrates (sugars and starches) into glucose, a simple sugar. Insulin also allows glucose to be absorbed by the bloodstream from the intestines, so the sugar can be used by muscles and tissues for energy or is stored in the liver until it is needed. Without insulin, glucose cannot be absorbed into the liver, muscles or tissues, and so remains in the bloodstream. High glucose levels in the blood can be damaging to the blood vessels and to various organs such as the heart, kidneys and eyes.

Some people tend to get diabetes in middle or later life. This is called maturity onset diabetes, and it is possible to have this for many months or even years, without realising it. Our modern lifestyle with little exercise and high-calorie foods has led to an epidemic of obesity. The fatter the body, the harder insulin has to work to control the blood glucose. High-sugar foods deluge the blood stream with waves of sugar, unlike what happens with the 'natural' hunter/gatherer diet of high fibre and slow-release complex sugars. All this puts a strain on the pancreas, which cannot produce enough insulin to keep the blood sugar under control. The blood sugar level goes up, and the person develops maturity onset diabetes.

Some people with maturity onset diabetes have no symptoms. Others feel extremely tired and very thirsty, lose weight and pass a lot of urine. Some women get continual vaginal thrush or skin boils. Because a high blood sugar level affects the lens of the eye, such that after a long time there are changes to the retina, opticians make the first diagnosis of diabetes in about 25 per cent of cases – in people who go to them because their eyesight has deteriorated.

There is often a strong genetic link with maturity onset diabetes. If either of your parents had diabetes in later life, it is sensible to have a fasting blood sugar check (see Chapter 9) once a year.

Some women develop diabetes when they are pregnant, only to find that the condition disappears when the baby is born. These 'gestational diabetics' are particularly at risk of developing diabetes later on, and again should be checked yearly.

Treatment

To avoid maturity onset diabetes, one should avoid obesity. Often if a person loses weight, her sugar level comes back under control.

Unfortunately, diabetes is a risk factor for cardiovascular disease, so diabetics should stop smoking, take up exercise and make efforts to lower their cholesterol (see Chapter 4). There is a variety of medications for diabetes, which can be prescribed by your doctor. Increasingly, maturity onset diabetics are being prescribed insulin injections in an effort to maximise good sugar control, thus minimising the long-term effects of the disease on blood vessels.

Anaemia

Anaemia is a condition in which the blood does not have enough red cells. It can occur for a number of reasons, all of which can be investigated by having blood tests done. Anaemia can make you feel tired all the time and short of breath.

Iron-deficient anaemia

The most common cause of anaemia in women is heavy periods. Vegetarians especially have great difficulty getting enough iron to replace the blood loss each month.

If a woman has iron-deficient anaemia, but does not have heavy periods, it indicates that there is blood loss from another source. This is usually the gut – a person could have piles, or more rarely a polyp, a gastric ulcer, or even cancer of the bowel.

Sometimes iron-deficient anaemia is simply the result of a poor diet. Occasionally, though, it could be because iron is not being absorbed from the gut properly, as in people with coeliac disease.

Vitamin B12 deficiency

Vitamin B12 is made in the gut and is needed to make red blood cells. In the old days, before B12 was discovered, a B12 deficiency was called 'pernicious anaemia' because it could not be treated. There is a familial link, and it is more common in people with blue eyes who go prematurely grey. A blood test can measure the level of B12, and treatment is with an injection every three months.

Folate deficiency

Folic acid is another chemical needed to make red blood cells. It is also given to pregnant women to lower the risk of spina bifida in babies.

Chapter 9

Examinations and investigations

About 75 per cent of menopausal woman seek information from their GP or primary care nurse about the menopause. Some women have a specific symptom or sign that is worrying them and which they wish to discuss. It may be a breast lump, or feelings of a prolapse (something 'coming down'), or very irregular vaginal bleeding. Women may feel non-specifically tired and unwell, and may wonder whether they are anaemic, or have an underactive thyroid, or are becoming diabetic. Most women just want to check that what they are experiencing is normal.

When you go to see your GP about any aspect of your health, he or she will want to know the 'history' of your complaint. So it is worth thinking beforehand about exactly what changes you have noticed, and making a note of them – if possible with the dates when they occurred. It is also valuable to write down what information you want from the consultation, so that you don't forget any important questions that you want to ask. If your symptoms are about the menopause, the GP might ask you about the following:

- the frequency and length of your periods over the last year
- any other symptoms (hot flushes, sleeplessness, etc.)
- what contraception you are using
- any problems with your bladder or bowels (e.g. incontinence, prolapse)
- any noticeable lumps in the breast
- when you last had a smear or mammogram
- what medications you are taking (including over-the-counter preparations such as St John's Wort – see Chapter 6)

- any past medical conditions of significance (e.g. deep vein thrombosis after pregnancy, breast cancer, chemotherapy)
- smoking and alcohol consumption; height and weight.

Physical examinations

It may be that the GP will have no need to examine you at all, if you have had a recent blood pressure check and if your reason for the appointment was mainly to get information. If you have a concern about particular symptoms, however, a physical examination may be necessary.

If you have discovered a breast lump, the doctor will want to examine your whole body, for example, to check for swollen lymph nodes (glands under the armpits and above the collar bones).

If you consult your doctor about urinary or faecal incontinence, an examination of the pelvic area will be necessary, both externally and internally. The doctor will need to see how relaxed your pelvic floor muscles are and whether your uterus is actually falling down into your vagina, or is even protruding from it (uterine prolapse). It is also important to check for pelvic masses, such as ovarian cysts or large fibroids of the uterus (see Chapters 2 and 8), that may be pressing on the pelvic organs and pushing them out. If you require a cervical smear this can be done at the same time.

If you think you may need to be examined, it is best to wear simple, loose-fitting clothes that are easy to get on and off. If you need a smear, you may feel more comfortable wearing a loose skirt, so you can keep it on and not feel so naked. You can either bring a friend or relative with you, or ask for a nurse or surgery staff to act as a chaperone during any intimate examination by a doctor.

Preliminary investigations performed by a GP

Depending on your symptoms or concerns, certain initial tests can by performed by your GP to determine whether further investigation is needed, perhaps in a specialist clinic.

Blood tests

When appropriate, hormone levels can be measured in women under 45 who have symptoms that may be menopausal (for more about premature menopause, see Chapter 1). However, blood tests may not be appropriate – if a woman is over 45 and is having classic menopausal symptoms, there is no point in measuring her hormones, as there will be no doubt that her symptoms are being caused by the menopause. (For more about hormonal changes at the menopause, see Chapter 1.)

Other blood tests that may be appropriate, depending on the symptoms, are:

- full blood count to check for anaemia
- thyroid function tests
- fasting blood glucose (no food after midnight, and only water to drink, with the blood test at 9am next morning), to exclude diabetes mellitus.

Mid-stream urine test

If a woman is having incontinence problems, the most likely explanation is a urinary tract infection (cystitis). Sometimes, if they have never had cystitis before, women do not realise they have got a bladder infection. Usually, however, you will know, as you will experience pain or burning when passing urine and will need to urinate much more often than usual, including getting up in the night to pass urine frequently. There may also be blood in the urine. With a severe urinary infection, women can feel systemically unwell (unwell throughout their body), as if they have flu. If symptoms of cystitis are present, a 'mid-stream' urine sample may be collected and sent to the laboratory. (It needs to be mid-stream because, when urinating, the first urine usually picks up skin bacteria and vaginal secretions from the skin around the opening to the bladder, which contaminate the urine and can give a confusing bacteriology result. So it is best to start to urinate, then stop after three seconds, then catch the next bit of urine in the specimen pot.)

The laboratory will investigate what bacteria is causing the infection, and will test for sugar to exclude the possibility of diabetes.

Breast investigations

Some breast tests, such as mammography, are routine screening procedures. They are either performed at your local hospital or at a screening mobile unit that may come to rural areas at a pre-arranged time. If you cannot make the appointment that you are given, call to make a new one. Breast awareness (see box) can be taught to you by your primary care nurse at your doctor's surgery. Breast cyst aspiration (see below) can be performed by a GP, although some prefer to send all women to a 'one-stop' breast clinic, where they can have the cyst or lump aspirated and wait to be told the result.

Breast awareness

All women should examine their breasts once a month, preferably just after their period, when the breasts are least lumpy. This way they will get used to knowing how their breasts feel and will be able to detect any change.

You should look for changes in shape, skin changes, any leaking from the nipples or any lumps that you have not noticed before. Breast tissue extends up to under the arms, so you should also feel from the breasts up into the armpits. It is easier to feel for changes with the soft pads of your fingers rather than the fingertips. Many women fear feeling their breasts, in case they find something suspicious, but you should remember that early detection of problems is crucial, as treatment is much more effective if it is commenced at an early stage. Never delay having anything unusual investigated because you are frightened to seek help, or think that you may be wasting the doctor's time.

You should see your GP if you notice any of the following:

- a breast lump
- indrawing (pulling in) of the nipple
- bloody discharge from the nipple
- change in the skin of the breast so it becomes puckered (coarse and bumpy, like the skin of an orange).

Mammography

A mammogram is an X-ray of the breasts, used to look for abnormalities and changes in the appearance of breast tissue. Very small breast cancers can be picked up using mammography long before the stage that anyone could feel them, and the cure rate from very early breast cancer is over 90 per cent. All women from the age of 50 to 64 are entitled and encouraged to attend for mammograms, and there is an automatic recall for these women every three years. Any woman over the age of 64 is entitled to request a mammogram.

The breasts are put between a firm table and a plate and are squashed slightly so that a good X-ray picture is obtained. This can feel slightly uncomfortable. Women who are on HRT or still have their own pre-menopausal hormones have 'denser' breasts than women who are not taking HRT and those who are post-menopausal. This means that the X-ray pictures look whiter, so it is harder to pick out tiny white dots of calcium, which might be early signs of cancer.

The way the screening service is organised will vary from area to area. Generally, each general practice in a given area will be visited in turn by the local breast screening mobile unit every three years. This means that not every woman is called to attend for a mammogram as soon as she is 50 years old. Ask at your surgery if you are concerned that you have not had an appointment. For more information, see *www.cancerscreening.nhs.uk/breastcreening/breastawareness.html*.

Cyst aspiration/aspiration biopsy

A cyst is a fluid-filled sac in the body. Cysts of the breast are extremely common, and they can be very painful if they have grown quickly and the fluid in the sac is under pressure. If you have a lump in your breast your GP may 'aspirate' the cyst in the surgery, or refer you to a specialist clinic for an aspiration biopsy. The doctor puts a fine needle through the skin straight into the cyst and sucks out with a syringe the fluid inside the cyst to completely empty it. The fluid may look green, yellow, clear or brown. If this is done by your GP, and the fluid contains blood or no fluid was aspirated, he or she will refer you to a breast clinic to have the lump investigated further. Fluid from the cyst should be sent to the laboratory for a cytology examination (when cells are looked at under the micro-scope to see if they are cancerous) to rule out any abnormal cells.

The advantage of having this procedure at a 'one-stop' hospital breast clinic is that you can have the cyst aspirated and an answer from the pathologist within about half an hour. The disadvantage is that you may have to wait several weeks for the appointment. Your

GP might be able to perform the procedure immediately, but then you both have to wait about a week for the results to come back from the laboratory. The 'one-stop' cytology is not as accurate as routine cytology, so if the pathologist thinks there are abnormal cells he or she might want to take a second, larger specimen with another needle, and prepare proper slides to make a firm diagnosis. This can take another seven to ten days of waiting.

Ultrasound scans

If breast cysts are suspected, sometimes ultrasound is used. Sound waves from a probe on the skin can produce a picture of the breast, and the cysts 'echo-located'. Sometimes cysts can be aspirated (see above) with the help of ultrasound location – the ultrasound picture means that the needle can be inserted at the exact spot where the cyst is.

Investigation and assessment of urinary incontinence

It is a brave woman who admits to incontinence. Anonymous postal surveys have indicated that at least one in ten women over 50 years experiences some degree of urinary incontinence, but only a tiny minority seek help from their GPs. Many women first experience urinary incontinence during pregnancy, when the elastic muscles of the pelvic floor are stretched and distorted by the weight of the huge pregnant uterus. Childbirth itself, or the method of delivery, can further destroy the muscles that keep the pelvic floor up in the pelvis, as well as the muscles (sphincters) that encircle the bladder and anus, keeping them closed until we want to open them (see Chapter 8 for more about pelvic floor laxity). After childbirth, with the help of pelvic floor exercises most women recover.

At the menopause, the drop in the levels of oestrogen allows the pelvic floor muscles to sag and the orifices to loosen, often resulting in **stress incontinence** – involuntary loss of urine on coughing, sneezing or laughing. This can be helped by local oestrogen treatment, pelvic floor exercises, or surgery. **Urge incontinence** – an involuntary loss of urine which may occur with the sudden urge to urinate – responds well to pelvic floor exercises (see Chapter 8).

Sometimes incontinence is not caused by pelvic floor sagging, but is due to an irritable, overactive bladder that just doesn't have the full capacity of a normal bladder. If this is the case, there are highly effective drugs that can relax the bladder wall muscles, so allowing greater filling and less urinary urgency. An 'overactive' bladder is known as **detrusor instability**.

The investigative tests for bladder problems are primarily to identify what has gone wrong, so the correct treatment can be offered. There are also tests to determine the severity of the incontinence. For some people there may be several elements to the problem, and they may therefore need several different approaches in their treatment. The GP will want to examine you, and may ask you to do the pad test or the frequency/volume chart (see below) before referring you to a continence clinic. And, as mentioned earlier in this chapter, he or she will also wish to exclude the possibility of a urinary infection (cystitis).

Assessing the degree of incontinence

Pad test

The International Continence Society has produced guidelines for a standardised one-hour pad test to provide objective demonstration of urinary leakage in order to reach the diagnosis of urinary incontinence. This is a simple non-invasive test for urinary incontinence. A pad is weighed and then worn for an hour. If the pad weight has increased by more than 2 grams over one hour of normal physical activity, it is considered significant. A weight gain of more than 10 grams in an hour is described as severe urinary incontinence.

Frequency and volume chart

This method provides very useful information about the volume of liquid drunk and excreted. The woman is asked to provide a chart of how much she drinks in a day, with the times and the volumes of the drinks. She also has to measure the volume of her urine, again recording the times.

Urinary flow measurements

A normal functional bladder voids 300 to 500mls of urine at one time. A measurement of urinary flow can be combined with measuring any urine left in the bladder at the end of urination ('residual urine volume'), which then provides information about how well the bladder empties.

The maximum urine flow rate (which can be determined by, for example, measuring the amount urinated into a measuring jug every second) is very dependent on the volume voided, and can be accurately measured only in volumes over 150mls. It is interesting to note that urine flow rates are higher in women than men for any comparable volume in the bladder.

Urinary flow is dependent on a number of factors. The muscles around the bladder contract to squeeze it, while the sphincter muscles that usually keep the bladder tightly shut have to relax. Problems can arise with either of these functions. Similarly, if the urethra (the tube down which urine passes from the bladder) is too narrow the urinary flow can be impeded. A prolonged, intermittent flow, with the patient straining to try to achieve bladder emptying, would suggest that this is the problem.

Tests for the causes of incontinence

The following tests are performed in specialist urodynamic laboratories in hospitals.

Cystometry

This is an invasive investigation of the structure and pressure-flow of the urinary tract, and measures pressure in the abdomen and in the bladder at the same time. It requires a 'pressure transducer' (a sensor that takes pressure and turns it into an electrical impulse that is then sent to a machine) to be threaded into the bladder, and another into either the rectum or vagina, to measure the abdominal pressure. If urinary leakage occurs on coughing and there is an associated rise in abdominal pressure but with no abnormal bladder activity, then urodynamic stress incontinence is diagnosed. This may be helped by surgery.

Video urodynamics

Video urodynamics (also known as video cytourethrography) allows the structure and pressure-flow of the urinary tract to be observed visually. A special contrast medium (rather like salt water) is put into the bladder with a catheter during cystometry, and the bladder is screened throughout the procedure, so that direct pictures of how the bladder behaves can be obtained. This method provides extra information about the shape of the bladder and the position of the bladder neck to the pubic arch. It can also show if there is reflux – urine going backwards up the ureters (the tubes that bring urine from the kidneys to the bladder). However, it is more costly than cystometry, in terms of time and equipment used, and does involve a dose of radiation for the patient. For most women it does not have an appreciable advantage over plain cystometry.

Neurological investigations

The normal coordinated functions of the bladder and urethra are controlled by a complex set of nerve reflexes, both in the spine and locally around the bladder. If it is thought likely that a problem in the functioning of these nerves is causing the incontinence, nerve conduction studies can be performed by recording electrical impulses generated by the nerves around the bladder and spinal cord.

Ultrasound

Ultrasound provides a non-invasive way of looking at the urinary tract over time without exposing the woman to any radiation, unlike video urodynamics, as it uses sound waves. Ultrasound is often used to look at the bladder after a woman has urinated to see whether there is a pool of stagnant urine left in the bladder after urination ('post-micturition residual volume'). This test is particularly relevant for women who have trouble passing water or who are incontinent when their bladder is full (**'overflow incontinence'**).

Cystourethroscopy

In this procedure, the woman is given a general anaesthetic and a tiny flexible fibre-optic instrument is passed up her urethra into her bladder, so the surgeon can see the inside of the urethra and bladder, and the openings of the ureters into the bladder. Sometimes the urethra becomes narrow ('stenosed'), and it can be gently widened by this process. In these cases a therapeutic dilatation can be done at the same time as the investigation, to correct the obstruction.

Tests for osteoporosis

It is agreed that mass screening of all women after the menopause for bone density, sometimes known as 'densitometry', is not necessary. However, 'high risk' groups should be screened – the National Osteoporosis Society* has criteria.

Dual-energy X-ray absorptiometry (DEXA) scans

These scans generally use X-rays at two different wavelengths to separate and identify soft tissue and bone. The process is therefore called dual-energy X-ray absorptiometry, or DEXA. This technique can accurately measure the mineral density of the bone, and is considered to be the 'gold standard' method for testing for osteoporosis at the spine and hip. In order to reduce the risks of an excess of radiation from repeated X-rays, bone scans are usually repeated only after about three years, although a second scan may be given one-and-a-half or two years after a new treatment has been started, to measure its effects. The advantage of blood sample measurements of bone markers (see Chapter 11) is that changes can be detected within four to six months of starting treatment.

Single-energy X-ray absorptiometry is commonly used for wrist scans. This involves a lower radiation dose, but only gives you information from one site, so may be a less accurate indication of the bone density overall. See Chapter 3 for more about DEXA.

Ultrasound scans

Ultrasound systems are being developed to measure heel bone. The heel bone was chosen for this method because it fits easily into the small machine. The machines used have the advantage of being portable and not using X-rays, but they need further testing before they are used more widely. They are also not so accurate as a DEXA, but do not expose the patient to any radiation. The machine is portable, so can be used to measure frail people in the community, such as those in an old people's home, rather than making them travel long distances to a specialist hospital centre. The main role of these systems is to help identify men and women at high risk of osteoporosis, and exclude those at low risk from years of unnecessary treatment, rather than being used to diagnose the condition or follow up women on treatment.

Blood or urine tests

In the future it may be possible to diagnose osteoporosis from a blood or urine test, by looking at chemicals associated with bone build-up or breakdown. Such a test should be able to detect changes such as response to treatment much more quickly (and safely) than bone scans. These bone 'markers' have been identified in the laboratory but are not yet available for routine use. See Chapter 11 for more details.

Examination of the uterus and endometrium

Taking HRT alters the risk of problems in the endometrium (the lining of the uterus). Various tests, described below, can be performed to look at the thickness of the endometrium and at its cells, to see whether they are normal, pre-cancerous or cancerous. Usually these tests are done if the woman's periods have become very heavy, or very irregular, or if she has had a postmenopausal bleed (a bleed after one year of not bleeding). It is very common to have these tests, and very uncommon to find any abnormality. The reason that these investigations are performed frequently is that early diagnosis of uterine cancer leads to a very high (over 95 per cent) cure rate. The first test is usually a scan.

Ultrasound scans

An ultrasound scan of the uterus is usually done from within your vagina, but can also be done through your stomach wall. It will look at the uterus and the ovaries. It looks not only at the endometrium thickness (the thicker the endometrium, the higher the risk of abnormal cells), but also checks for fibroids or cysts on the ovaries.

Biopsy

A biopsy, or small sample of tissue, may need to be taken from the lining of the uterus. A biopsy is usually done without an anaesthetic by passing a fine tube through the neck of the uterus and obtaining the tissue with gentle suction. The procedure is similar to having a smear test, but slightly more painful for the few seconds of the suction. You may have some period-like pain during and after the procedure. In some cases, however, the biopsy is obtained under general anaesthetic, usually as a day case, and may be called a dilatation and curettage or 'D&C'.

Hysteroscopy

A hysteroscopy is a direct viewing of the inside of the uterus. It involves passing a fine fibre-optic instrument through the neck of the uterus and can be done either with or without a general anaesthetic.

Smear tests

It is important to continue to have regular smears after the menopause, and most general practices notify their patients when a smear is due every three years until screening ends at the age of 65. At the time of writing there is some controversy about the age at which screening for cervical cancer should finish. Some suggest the age should be reduced to 55 years, on the grounds that most cervical abnormalities are found in women below this age, and that cervical screening is more uncomfortable postmenopausally, as the vagina gets dryer. It is also technically more difficult to get a good cell sample, as there are fewer cervical cells to harvest. However, it is vital to continue having smears if:

- you have had an abnormality in the past
- you have a new sexual partner
- your current sexual partner gets a new sexual partner as well as you.

Chapter 10

Phytoestrogens and SERMs

In Australia in the 1940s a huge flock of sheep unexpectedly did not produce lambs in the spring. This infertility was inexplicable because the rams had a proven track record of reproducing, so a vet was called in to investigate. The ewes had been grazing on a species of red clover which was rich in a phytoestrogen. Phytoestrogens are natural plant molecules that have a weak oestrogenic effect on any mammal which eats the plants. If huge amounts are eaten, the effect can be significant. Red clover contains formononetin, a molecule that is converted to daidzein, the active phytoestrogen, during fermentation in the stomach. The animals were found to have cystic ovaries, stimulated by excessive amounts of phytoestrogen. After the farmer stopped the flock eating the clover, the ewes returned to their normal fecundity.

There has been an upsurge of interest in these natural substances and their effect on the human population. Many people are looking for dietary ways of improving their fitness and lowering their risk of disease, and phytoestrogens may present some solutions. Many questions about them have not been answered yet, but trials are going on at present. It appears that phytoestrogens can reduce the incidence of hot flushes in menopausal women, lower serum cholesterol, and possibly lower the risk of prostate cancer, breast cancer and cardio-vascular disease: all major killers in the over-50 age group, where any change in the mortality rates would have a significant impact.

What are phytoestrogens?

Phytoestrogens are chemical compounds found in cereals, legumes, citrus fruits and grasses. There are many classes of phytoestrogens, but isoflavones and lignans have been studied the most. Of the thousand or so isoflavones in plants, only a small number have oestrogenic activity, and four are found in the human diet: daidzein, genistein, formononetin and biochanin. These four molecules are so close in shape to an oestrogen molecule that they 'fool' the oestrogen receptor into activity. However, because they are not an exact fit, they do not have the power to activate the oestrogen receptor in quite the same way that a real oestrogen molecule has. It is rather like using a bent paper clip (the phytoestrogen) – rather than the key (the oestrogen molecule) – to open a lock (the oestrogen receptor).

Compounds with oestrogen-like activity and their common food sources

Phytoestrogen	Food source
lignans	vegetables, fruits, nuts, cereals, spices
isoflavones	soya, peas, clover, beans, spinach, fruits
chalcones	liquorice
flavones	beans, green vegetables, fruits, nuts
coumarins	cabbage, peas, spinach, liquorice
acyclics	hops (beer)

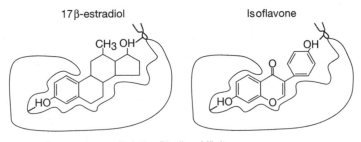

Relative Binding Affinity		
	ER-α	ER-β
Estradiol	100	100
Genistein	5	36

Figure 1   The oestrogen receptor

Red clover leaves contain 2 per cent by weight of isoflavones, and have all four oestrogenic isoflavones. Soya beans contain 0.2 per cent daidzein and genistein by weight. Beans form the staple diet of many people in Asian countries, who therefore consume significant amounts of isoflavones, whereas the typical Western diet contains less than one half-cup serving of beans or peas per day.

The most investigated molecules of the isoflavone group are genistein, daidzein and equol. Soya contains genistin, the glycosylated form of genistein. It becomes oestrogenically active only after it has been absorbed through the gut, where bacteria alter its molecular structure.

Lignans are widespread in the plant world, where they are the building blocks of lignin in the plant cell walls. A rich source of lignans is linseed (flax seed). Again, when they are eaten, the gut flora remove the glucose groups and methyl groups to form molecules structurally similar to estradiol.

The effects of phytoestrogens on humans

When eaten, phytoestrogens are absorbed though the gut and then circulate though the bloodstream. They behave like very weak oestrogen molecules at oestrogen receptor sites around the body. The effect oestrogen has on the body is over a thousand times greater than that of these molecules, so their effects are minuscule, but over many years on a daily basis they do appear to have a small effect.

Strength of phytoestrogens	
If estradiol is assigned a potency (strength) of	100.0
genistein has a relative potency of	0.084
equol has a relative potency of	0.0161
daidzein has a relative potency of	0.013

Phytoestrogens also appear to actively simulate certain effects on oestrogen receptors, while inhibiting other oestrogen effects in other tissues. This is rather confusing, but is similar to the effect of tamoxifen (see 'Tamoxifen', below). This may also explain some of the rather confusing findings that appear to be emerging about phytoestrogens, and the difficulties in designing medical trials.

Menopausal symptoms

As was pointed out in Chapters 2 and 7, the traditional Japanese diet has a high amount of soya bean, and it is estimated that the average Japanese person consumes up to 200mg of isoflavones per day. In contrast the diet of the average Londoner contains 30–60mg of isoflavones. Japanese women have a very low rate of hot flushes (as few as 5–10 per cent) compared with menopausal women in the UK, where up to 80 per cent complain to their GPs about them. Of course, as has been explored in Chapter 2, cultural factors could also be responsible for this, with women in Japan more reluctant to talk about their symptoms, but the difference has stimulated medical research into the area.

There have been several studies looking at dietary supplementation of isoflavones in menopausal women. A placebo-controlled study over a 12-week period showed a significant decrease in menopausal symptoms. A similar study with a four-week time scale showed no effect, which would imply that women need to eat phytoestrogen-rich diets for at least six weeks before any effect can be observed. In an Australian study, 50 postmenopausal women were treated with red clover leaf extract in a double-blind, cross-over trial (one in which neither the volunteers nor the investigators know which are the active ingredients being tested and which are ones that look identical but do not contain the active ingredient). The study found a correlation between daidzein levels and decreased menopausal symptoms, but there was no overall difference between the treatment and placebo groups.

Breast cancer

Given that phytoestrogens seem to have a weakly oestrogenic effect, one might expect phytoestrogen eaters to have a higher incidence of breast cancer, just like long-term hormone replacement therapy (HRT) users. At present this does **not** seem to be so. In fact, epidemiological studies seem to show that a phytoestrogen-rich diet lowers the risk of breast cancer. It is not actually clear at present whether this is because of an anti-oestrogen effect at the tissue level, similar to that of substances like tamoxifen (see 'Tamoxifen', below). Another explanation is that women on largely vegetarian diets have a lower fat and meat intake, and so are eating fewer carcinogens (it is thought that a diet high in animal fat is slightly more carcinogenic). All the studies done so far can be criticised in the way they were set up: crucially, they did not distinguish between pre- and postmenopausal breast cancer.

Endometrial cancer

Given the oestrogenic effect of phytoestrogens, it might be thought that women taking phytoestrogen-enriched diets could be at greater risk of endometrial (womb) cancer, similar to women taking tamoxifen for a long time, or unopposed oestrogens as HRT. At present, however, there are no reported increased risks associated with phytoestrogens, and the incidence of endometrial cancer in Japan is lower than that in the UK, even though Japanese women have fewer children, which should put them at a higher risk. This also points to a possible anti-oestrogenic effect at the endometrial level, or it could be because of a selective oestrogen receptor modulator effect (see section on SERMs, below). The SERM raloxifene acts in this way with no increased risk of endometrial cancer.

As mentioned above, it is known that the fewer the number of pregnancies, the higher the risk of endometrial cancer, so women at greatest risk are those who have never had children. However, there are other variables. Fatter women have a much higher risk of breast and endometrial cancer than women of a normal or thin body mass. This is because obese women have higher circulating levels of estradiol produced in their fatty tissue. In Japan, obesity is not as generalised as it is in the Western world, so it is difficult to control for this factor.

Bowel and prostate cancers

Bowel and prostate cancers are a major, and increasing, source of illness and death in the over-50 age group, especially in Western countries. The phytoestrogen genistein has been shown to inhibit the enzyme tyrosine kinase, which is involved in the control of cell division, cell cycle regulation and cell survival. Laboratory studies have shown that various cancer cell lines from breast, bowel and prostate have all been inhibited by genistein. These effects are independent of any anti-oestrogen receptor effect. In animal models, soya bean proteins have been shown to prevent prostatitis and prostatic dysplasia (the stage before cells become cancerous). So at present phytoestrogens appear to be good for men as well as for women.

Osteoporosis

Japanese women have a lower incidence of hip fractures than Caucasian women, and osteoporosis is lower in Asian women in Asia than Western women in the same environment. It is hard to say, however, what the reason for this is, as the roles played by diet, genes, exercise, smoking, alcohol, sunshine exposure, number of pregnancies, breastfeeding and hysterectomy rates are very difficult to tease apart. Genistein has been shown to prevent bone loss in rats which have had their ovaries surgically removed.

A study of women taking isoflavone for a period of 12 weeks did not show any effect on bone turnover, but that might be because it was not a long enough period for the isoflavones to have a measurable effect on bone metabolism.

Fats and heart disease

Heart disease is the biggest cause of death in the over-60 age group for both men and women in the UK. Postmenopausal women who are not on HRT rapidly lose their protection from heart attacks and strokes because of the falling levels of oestrogen. Arterial disease, in which the arteries become furred up with fatty deposits known as plaques, is caused by many different factors: lifestyle (smoking, obesity, high fat intake), genetics, diabetes mellitus, high blood pressure, kidney failure, an early menopause and inherited high blood fats. Preventive health care involves trying to reduce all these risk factors (see Chapters 4 and 7).

Oestrogens in HRT and tamoxifen have been shown to decrease low-density lipoproteins (LDL), which are thought to be the dangerous form of cholesterol (see Chapter 4) as far as arterial disease is concerned. Soya has been shown to lower total cholesterol, and possibly raise the 'good' high-density lipoproteins (HDL) levels by 12 to 34 per cent in people with a high cholesterol.

Selective Oestrogen Receptor Modulators (SERMs)

About 80 per cent of menopausal women in the UK are *not* on hormone replacement therapy. Women choose not to take HRT for a variety of reasons (see Chapters 5 and 6). Most women feel that the menopause is a normal milestone in women's lives and should not be medicalised. Other women would like something for the symptoms of hot flushes but find the realities of HRT sometimes worse than the menopausal symptoms for which they were taking it. The vast majority of women choose to put up with the discomforts of the menopause rather than increase their risk of breast cancer by taking HRT. The absolutely perfect HRT that would improve bones, lower risks of strokes and heart attacks, lower cholesterol, stop women getting Alzheimer's disease but not give them breast cancer or clots in their legs has not been invented yet. This would be the perfect 'designer' HRT.

Tamoxifen

Tamoxifen has been used to help prevent the spread of breast cancer, in affected women, for at least three decades. Millions of women have been treated with tamoxifen. It always used to be thought of as an anti-oestrogen – i.e., that it counteracted the effect of oestrogen on tissues. This explained why it was effective against breast cancer as breast tumours are usually hormone sensitive. The surprising thing about tamoxifen is that women who have been on it for some time have a better bone density than women who have not taken it. If it truly worked as an anti-oestrogen women who take it would be expected to have worse bone density, increasing their risk of osteoporosis. The other surprising thing about tamoxifen is that it appears to stimulate the endometrium (the lining of the womb). This can sometimes lead to long-term users of tamoxifen experiencing irregular bleeding or even womb cancer. Again, if tamoxifen was simply acting as an anti-oestrogen it should not be stimulating the lining of the womb. These somewhat contradictory effects of tamoxifen show that it is not acting in a simple way on our bodies at all. In some tissues (such as the breast) the molecule works as an anti-oestrogen, and in others (such as bones and the endometrium) it acts rather like the oestrogen molecule itself.

What are SERMs?

Selective Oestrogen (Estrogen in the USA, hence the acronym) Receptor Modulators were launched in 1998 as a new class of drugs in the HRT market.

The apparently paradoxical effect of tamoxifen in women has inspired drug companies to do further research into its interesting properties, in order to tweak the molecule in such a way that it would be an 'ideal HRT'. This idea of selectively sparking off some oestrogen receptors in the body and not others has given rise to SERMs.

Raloxifene (Evista) is the first SERM on the British market. In some oestrogen receptors the raloxifene molecule is embraced, to stimulate the receptor, while in others it blocks the effect.

The early evidence from the use of raloxifene shows that it improves bone density, lowers serum cholesterol and does not effect the womb. There is no increased risk of stimulation of the lining of the womb or womb cancer. Similarly it does not stimulate breast tissue and women taking raloxifene have a 30 per cent lower incidence of breast cancer than women on a placebo.

Are SERMs too good to be true?

While it might appear that SERMs are a designer HRT, the one disadvantage known so far is that they cause the same slight increased rate of venous thrombosis, clots in the legs, as real oestrogens. This is a very small risk but one women should know about. Moreover, data on whether they lead to a higher risk of heart attacks and strokes is not available yet.

A major drawback of using raloxifene is that, ironically, it can cause hot flushes, and it does not help the immediate menopausal symptoms which motivate women to take HRT in the first place. At present SERMs are designed for women over 60 who want to stay on HRT but wish to lower their risk of breast cancer.

Chapter 11

The future

This chapter looks briefly at treatments or drugs that are already at the research stage, so it is likely that they will be in the public domain within five years. Some of them are surgical and others medical, but they are all relevant to women going through the menopause.

Vertebroplasty

An osteoporotic fracture of a vertebra can be excruciatingly painful. A vertebroplasty is an injection though the skin and muscle of the back into the vertebral bone that has been fractured. When the needle is in the fractured bone, cement is squirted in though the needle to stabilise the bone fragments. Vertebroplasty can be an extremely effective procedure for pain relief, providing improvement in 80–90 per cent of appropriately selected cases. The early treatment of fractures by vertebroplasty remains controversial. It has been found that after six months there is no significant difference between people treated with vertebroplasty and those who underwent conventional treatments with medical advice and good pain relief. Moreover, vertebroplasty is very expensive for the NHS, because it requires a highly skilled doctor to do the procedure and a screening room in the radiology department. Risks to the patient include bleeding or infection when the needle is introduced into the bone, leaking of cement beyond the vertebral walls and into the spinal canal, paraplegia, and cement going into blood vessels which can result in pulmonary emboli (clots of cement in the lungs) or brain, causing a stroke.

Some doctors have noticed that the vertebrae either side of the cemented one often fracture soon afterwards. There is uncertainty about whether the extra-firm cemented vertebra actually causes fractures of the others by its change in material compressability, or whether these vertebrae would have fractured anyway, because they are all so fragile.

It seems reasonable to advise patients to try six weeks of conventional medical treatment first before going in for vertebroplasty unless their pain cannot be satisfactorily controlled or their immobility from the pain is putting them at risk.

Kyphoplasty

In November 2003 the National Institute for Clinical Excellence (NICE) issued guidance that balloon kyphoplasty should not be used without the special consent of the patient, as it was felt that the benefits were insufficient to outweigh the risks. Balloon kyphoplasty differs from vertebroplasty in that a balloon is inserted into the fractured vertebra and gently pumped up to restore the original thickness of the squashed vertebral bone. Once the balloon is inflated, cement is injected in though the needle, so not only is the fracture stabilised by the cement, but the height of the vertebra is restored. Because the cement is injected into the balloon cavity, leakage of cement is less of a risk than it is in vertebroplasty. Kyphoplasty has to be performed under a general anaesthetic, so it is much more expensive in terms of resources, with an operating theatre, anaesthetist, nurses and a trained neurosurgeon needed. There is also the added risk of death from a general anaesthetic of one in 10,000. The real outcome in pain relief and mobility improvement between vertebroplasty and kyphoplasty has not yet been quantified in controlled medical trials, which are at present ongoing.

Bone markers to measure bone turnover

The human skeleton responds to wear and tear by 'bone remodelling', that is the bone resorbs (or breaks down) parts and replaces worn bits. The rate of bone replacement closely follows that of bone resorption. All the drugs that stop osteoporosis by preventing bone resorption also suppress bone synthesis. So if a measure of bone synthesis is used, it is a good marker that bone turnover is responding to treatment. It is a much faster measure than a DEXA scan (see Chapter 3), where not much change is seen within two years. Bone markers will show a difference within three to four months of therapy. This is useful because the person taking the therapy – as well as the medical professionals overseeing it – can see if it is working.

There are many different bone markers. One that has been used experimentally in Oxford and is now being used generally is P1NP (N-teloptide of type 1 collagen).

The measurement should be performed on a simple blood specimen (but it has to get to the laboratory the same day, which can be a problem in rural GP practices).

It should be done:

- before treatment starts, to get a baseline figure
- after three to four months of treatment, to see if treatment is working
- yearly to check bone turnover.

The disadvantage of bone markers is that they cannot be interpreted if there has been a recent fracture, which is often when therapy is started.

The advantage of bone markers is that a change can be seen so soon after treatment. A bone marker test costs the NHS about £5, as opposed to £50 for a DEXA scan. This could free up DEXA scans for more appropriate use, i.e. for new referrals rather than rescanning present users. It is a better predictor of fracture risk than bone densitometry, because it gives an indication of bone quality.

Bisphosphonates

Bisphosphonates (see also Chapter 3) are a class of drugs used in the treatment of established osteoporosis and are a useful alternative to ovarian hormone therapy in postmenopausal women with osteoporosis. It is not known whether bisphosphonates are effective after five years of treatment. Very prolonged treatment may, in fact, not be beneficial. Bisphosphonates affect remodelling, thus preventing new bone forming (although preventing old bone being resorbed), so tiny microfractures accumulate that are not repaired, eventually resulting in weaker bone. Specialists are offering patients a 'drug holiday' after five years on a bisphosphonate, allowing the osteoblasts and osteoclasts to recover and remodel the cracks. Current research suggests that bone turnover is suppressed for at least 18 months after stopping alendronate, a bisphosphonate. By having annual bone marker turnover measurements, patients can be monitored to know when they should start treatment again after the holiday.

At present there are once-weekly preparations of bisphosphonate on the market. Ones in medical trials at present are other oral preparations that need be taken only once a month, and an infusion of bisphosphonate that lasts one year.

Teriparatide

Parathyroid hormone (PTH) and some of its fragments are important in bone formation. One fragment, teriparatide, has been engineered and patented, and has been shown to stimulate osteoblasts. It needs to be given by daily injection. In studies it has been shown to reduce vertebral and non-vertebral fragility fractures.

The disadvantage to the NHS is that the treatment is extremely expensive – the cost for 18 months of treatment is £5,316. The disadvantages to the patient are that they need to have daily injections, which could lead to some local irritation, nausea or diarrhoea.

The perfect designer HRT?

The magic molecule many researchers are looking for is the perfect Selective Oestrogen Receptor Modulator (SERM, see Chapter 10). It would be a molecule that protects women against breast cancer, heart disease, Alzheimer's and womb cancer, and yet stops hot flushes and gives women strong bones. Raloxifene has found some success, but because it can make hot flushes worse it is not useful for the perimenopausal women.

Ovarian conservation

Women go through the menopause because the ovaries run out of eggs. If some ovarian tissue were saved and frozen early on, to be reimplanted at the menopause, would women remain eternally youthful and healthy? Researchers are trying to freeze ovarian tissue from young girls who are about to undergo chemotherapy and/or radiotherapy, which would otherwise render them infertile and give them an early menopause. This research is at a very early phase, but might bring new hope for some young women in the next few years.

Glossary

acute vertebral collapse A drop in the height of the spinal column resulting from a break or fracture in the vertebrae of the spine; a typical sign of osteoporosis

amenorrhoea Absence of periods. The most common cause of amenorrhoea in women aged 15–45 is pregnancy; in women older than 45 it is the menopause

analgesia A method of pain relief

androgens Hormones (q.v.) present in men and women, but more so in men

angina Pain resulting from the heart muscle getting cramp when exercised, caused by inadequate blood supply (*see ischaemic heart disease*)

benign Non-cancerous. Benign lumps may grow but will not spread to other parts of the body or cause widespread damage

biopsy The removal of a small sample of tissue (e.g. from the lining of womb, or breast) to be looked at under a microscope in a laboratory

blood pressure A measurement of the pressure at which blood is flowing through the blood vessels. High levels can damage blood vessels and increase the risk of heart disease

bone mass and **bone mineral density** *See osteoporosis*

calcium A mineral found in the diet chiefly in milk and dairy products. It is required for healthy strong bones

cancer An abnormal proliferation of cells which may cause a lump (tumour) and may spread to other parts of the body, interfering with normal function

cardiovascular system The heart and blood vessels

cervical smear test See smear test

cervix The neck of the womb. Cervical smears are taken from the cells in this area

cholesterol One of the fats in the blood which is used to produce hormones and perform other vital functions. Excess levels in the blood may cause deposits which can block blood vessels and cause heart disease

collagen A protein produced in the body which helps make up living tissues, like bone and skin. It is slightly elastic, and in women, its properties can be changed by oestrogen (q.v.)

combined oral contraceptive Contraceptive pill combining oestrogen (q.v.) and normally a progestogen (q.v.)

cyst A fluid-filled sac found in any part of the body

cystitis Inflammation of the bladder causing painful urination

diabetes mellitus Insufficient production of the hormone insulin by the pancreas, to deal with glucose (sugar) from the diet. High blood levels of glucose result, which can be damaging for many parts of the body

deep vein thrombosis (DVT) A clot in the deep veins of the leg. Deep vein thrombosis can occur out of the blue, but it is more common if circulation of blood around the leg is slowed down for any reason. It can also occur during pregnancy and among women taking the oral contraceptive pill or HRT (q.v.)

dilatation and curettage (D&C) A 'scrape' performed under general anaesthetic to remove cells from the lining of the womb

discharge Abnormal or unusual fluid produced by a part of the body

dysmenorrhoea Painful periods

dyspareunia Painful sex

electrocardiogram (ECG) An electrical recording of the heart rhythms

endometrium The lining of the womb that is shed each month, causing a period

endometriosis A condition in which cells of the endometrium are found outside the womb (e.g. on the ovaries) and may cause pain, adhesions and cysts as they swell and bleed during periods

fibroids Thickened bulges of the muscular wall of the womb (myometrium) which cause a bump or protrusion. Fibroids can be on the outside of the womb, in the womb wall or projecting into the internal cavity of the womb. Most women over 40 have fibroids

follicle stimulating hormone (FSH) *See pituitary hormones*

heart attack *See ischaemic heart disease*

hormone A chemical produced by a gland which has an effect on other parts of the body

hormone replacement therapy (HRT) A medical treatment designed to restore the natural hormones produced by the ovary in the body to a level that were produced by that woman before her menopause. Combined HRT (oestrogen + progestogens) is used for women who still have wombs; oestrogen alone is used for those who have had total hysterectomies

hysterectomy Surgical removal of the womb (uterus). A total hysterectomy is removal of the whole womb, a subtotal hysterectomy leaves behind the cervix (q.v.). A hysterectomy can be performed from an incision in the low abdomen or through the vagina thus preventing an abdominal scar. It can also be removed using keyhole surgery with a laparoscope

hysteroscopy A fibre optic instrument used by a gynaecologist to look directly at the lining of the womb

incontinence Lack of urinary or faecal control

intrauterine contraceptive device (IUCD) and **intrauterine contraceptive system (IUCS)** A small plastic object that is inserted into the womb to provide contraception. An IUCD has copper wrapped round the core, which gives an added effect. The new levonorgestrel system (IUCS) has a progestogen (q.v.) in the core, which is released over many years

ischaemic heart disease Poor blood supply to the heart resulting from the furring up of the coronary arteries (the vessels that supply blood to the heart). The term can be used when a person is suffering from angina (q.v.) or from a myocardial infarction (a heart attack, when a blood clot blocks the blood flow to coronary artery), or both

kyphoplasty Surgical repair of a collapsed vertebra

laparoscope A small fibre optic instrument inserted into the abdominal cavity to enable a specialist to look around inside

lumbar The lower region of the back from the waist down to where the spine fits into the pelvic bones

lutenising hormone (LH) *See pituitary hormones*

malignant Cancerous

menopause The last menstrual period. If a women has not had a period for a year, she is defined as having gone through the menopause

menorrhagia Excessively heavy bleeding during periods

oestrogen A hormone produced by the ovaries which is responsible for female sexual characteristics. Levels fall after the menopause and are replaced in hormone replacement therapy (HRT, q.v.)

oestrogen receptors Special places in the tissue where the oestrogen molecule has been shown to be specifically attracted, like a key into a lock; they exist on the cells of the urethra, bladder, vagina and the muscles of the pelvic floor. Oestrogen can have an effect only on tissues that contain oestrogen receptors

oöphorectomy Surgical removal of the ovary (q.v.). If one ovary is removed, it is termed 'unilateral oöphorectomy'

osteoarthritis Wear and tear on a joint between two moving bones that often causes great pain. It is sometimes known as 'degenerative change', as it is a process that happens over many years

osteopenia A condition of low bone mineral density (i.e. not enough calcium in bones)

osteoporosis Loss of bone cells leading to brittle and weak bones which may cause pain and fractures; the loss accelerates after menopause

ovarian failure The failure of the ovaries to produce an egg each month. This happens naturally at the menopause, and is the cause of the menopause. It may occur after chemotherapy or radiotherapy to the abdomen, or after hysterectomy (q.v.) even if the ovaries are left behind

ovary The organ in the body that produces eggs. It also produces the oestrogen and progesterone hormones. Normally women have two ovaries

perimenopause About three to five years before a woman's periods actually cease forever, during which changes are slowly taking place in both the ovary and the pituitary hormones. Women begin to have symptoms of hot flushes, irritability and tiredness at this time

phytoestrogens Naturally occurring plant substances which, when eaten, act as weak oestrogens in the body

pituitary hormones A variety of chemical messengers or hormones secreted into the blood by the pituitary gland. Two hormones, the follicle stimulating hormone (FSH) and the luteinising hormone (LH) stimulate the ovary to produce an egg on a monthly cycle

polyps Benign little blobs of tissue, sometimes on the cervix or the endometrium, that usually just need to be pulled off by a trained gynaecologist or GP

postmenopausal bleeding Bleeding from the vagina which occurs a year (or longer) after all periods have stopped. It should be investigated by your GP

postmenopause The entire part of woman's life after she has gone through the menopause

progesterone A hormone produced from the cyst in the ovary after the egg has ripened and popped into the fallopian tube

progestogen Synthetic substance with an action in the body that mimics progesterone

prolapse The downward movement of any organ, usually the womb, owing to the weakening of its supporting structures such as ligaments and muscles. May be accompanied by weakness of the wall between the womb and the bladder (cystocele), or the wall between the womb and the rectum (rectocele)

pulmonary embolus (PE) A very serious, potentially fatal, condition in which a blood clot in the deep veins (DVT, q.v.) spreads from the lower leg to above the knee, or in the pelvic veins, and breaks off and travels to the lungs

Selective Oestrogen Receptor Modulators (SERMs) Molecules that act on some oestrogen receptors in the body. They help protect bone, and may also protect the breast, as they are based on the tamoxifen molecule, which is used to treat breast cancer

smear test The screening test for cervical cancer. A sample of cells is taken from the cervix with the use of a spatula or brush; the sample is examined under the microscope in a laboratory for pre-cancerous, treatable changes

systemic Affecting the whole body rather than a specific part of it

tachyphylaxis A condition in which the body gets used to the effect of a certain medicine so that subsequently bigger doses are needed to have an effect. This can occur with oestrogen implants with women requiring them more frequently

ultrasound A diagnostic technique which uses sound waves to bounce off internal organs and give an image on the screen which can be interpreted

uterus The womb

vagina The front passage which leads to the womb

Addresses and useful contacts

Action on Smoking and Health
102 Clifton Street
London EC2A 4HW
Tel: 020-7739 5902
Fax: 020-7613 0531
Email: enquiries@ash.org.uk
Website: www.ash.org.uk

Alcoholics Anonymous
PO Box 1
Stonebow House
Stonebow
York YO1 7NJ
Tel: (01904) 644026
Check your telephone directory for details of your local group

Alzheimer's Society
Gordon House
10 Greencoat Place
London SW1P 1PH
Tel: 020-7306 0606
Helpline: (0845) 300 0336
Fax: 020-7306 0808
Email: enquiries@alzheimers.org.uk
Website: www.alzheimers.org.uk

ASH Scotland
6 Frederick Street
Edinburgh EH2 2HB
Tel: 0131-225 4725
Fax: 0131-225 4759
Email:
ashscotland@ashscotland.org.uk
Website: www.ashscotland.org.uk

Breast Cancer Care
Kiln House
210 New Kings Road
London SW6 4NZ
Tel: 020-7384 2984
Helpline: (0808) 800 6000
(10am–5pm Mon to Fri)
Website: www.breastcancercare.org.uk

British Association of Nutritional Therapists (BANT)
27 Old Gloucester Street
London WC1N 3XX
Tel/Fax: (0870) 606 1284
Website: www.bant.org.uk

British Complementary Medicine Association (BCMA)
PO Box 5122
Bournemouth BH8 0WG
Tel: (0845) 345 5977
Email: info@bcma.co.uk
Website: www.bcma.co.uk

British Heart Foundation
14 Fitzhardinge Street
London W1H 6DH
Tel: 020-7935 0185
Heart Information Line:
(08450) 70 80 70
Fax: 020-7486 5820
Email: internet@bhf.org.uk
Website: www.bhf.org.uk

British Menopause Society
Website: www.the-bms.org

British Thyroid Foundation
PO Box 97
Clifford
Wetherby
West Yorkshire LS23 6XD
Tel: (0870) 770 7933
Website: www.btf-thyroid.org
Patient-led charitable organisation, run by
volunteers and thyroid sufferers in
conjunction with medical advisers

Cancer BACUP
3 Bath Place
Rivington Street
London EC2A 3JR
Tel: 020-7696 9003
Freephone: (0808) 800 1234
Fax: 020-7696 9002
Website: www.cancerbacup.org.uk

Cancer Research Campaign
PO Box 123
Lincoln's Inn Fields
London WC2A 3PX
Tel: 020-7009 8820
Fax: 020-7269 3100
Website: www.cancerresearchuk.org

Committee on Safety of Medicines
Market Towers
1 Nine Elms Lane
Vauxhall
London SW8 5NQ
Tel: 020-7084 2451
Fax: 020-7084 2493
Website:
www.mca.gov.uk/aboutagency/
regframework/csm/csmhome.htm

Continence Foundation
307 Hatton Square
16 Baldwins Gardens
London EC1N 7RJ
Tel: (0845) 345 0165
(9.30am–1pm Mon to Fri)
Email: continence-help@
dial.pipex.com
Website:
www.continencefoundation.org.uk
For leaflets, email with your address
details or write enclosing a large SAE

Depression Alliance
35 Westminster Road
London SE1 7JB
Tel: 020-7633 0557
Fax: 020-7633 0559
Website: www.depressionalliance.org

Depression Alliance Scotland
3 Grosvenor Gardens
Edinburgh EH12 5JU
Tel: 0131-467 3050
Fax: 0131-467 7701
Website:
www.depressionalliance.org/scotland/
Scotland_news.htm

Depression Alliance Wales
11 Plas Melin
Westbourne Road
Whitchurch
Cardiff CF4 2BT
Tel: 029-2069 2891
Fax: 029-2052 1774
Website: www.depressionalliance.
org/wales/index.htm

Diabetes UK
10 Parkway
London NW1 7AA
Tel: 020-7424 1000
Careline: (0845) 120 2960
Fax: 020-7424 1001
Email: info@diabetes.org.uk
Website: www.diabetes.org.uk

**Friends of the Western Buddhist
Order (FWBO)**
Communications Office
59 Roman Road
London E2 0QN
Tel: 020-8981 8000
Email: communications@fwbo.org
Website: www.fwbo.org
*For your nearest Buddhist Centre visit the
website*

Incontact
United House
North Road
London N7 9DP
Tel: (0870) 770 3246
Fax: (0870) 779 3249
Email: info@incontact.org
Website: www.incontact.org
*A membership organisation run by and for
people with bowel and bladder problems
and their carers*

**Institute of Complementary Medicine
(ICM)**
PO Box 194
London SE16 7QZ
Tel: 020-7237 5165
Fax: 020-7237 5175
Email: icm@icmedicine.co.uk
Website: www.icmedicine.co.uk

Menopause Amarant Trust
Tel helpline: (01293) 413000
(11am–6pm, Mon to Fri)
Website:
www.amarantmenopausetrust.org.uk

The Menopause Exchange
PO Box 205
Bushey
Herts WD23 1ZS
Tel: 020-8420 7245
Email: mexchange@btinternet.com

National Endometriosis Society
50 Westminster Palace Gardens
Artillery Row
London SW1P 1RR
Tel: 020-7222 2781
Fax: 020-7222 2786
Email: nes@endo.org.uk
Website: www.endo.org.uk

**National Institute for Clinical
Excellence**
MidCity Place
71 High Holborn
London WC1V 6NA
Tel: 020-7067 5800
Fax: 020-7067 5801
Email: nice@nice.nhs.uk
Website: www.nice.org.uk

NHS Direct
Tel: (0845) 46 47
Website: www.nhsdirect.nhs.uk

NHS Direct Scotland
Tel: (0845) 424 2424

National Institute of Medical Herbalists (NIMH)
56 Longbrook Street
Exeter EX4 6AH
Email:
nimh@ukexeter.freeserve.co.uk
Website: www.nimh.org.uk

National Osteoporosis Society (NOS)
Camerton
Bath BA2 0PJ
Tel: (01761) 471771
(general enquiries)
Tel: (0845) 450 0230
(medical queries)
Fax: (01761) 471104
Email: info@nos.org.uk
Website: www.nos.org.uk

Natural Health Advisory Service
PO Box 268
Lewes
East Sussex BN7 1QN
Tel: (01273) 487366
Fax: (01273) 487576
Email:
enquiries@naturalhealthas.com
Website: www.wnas.org.uk

Quitline
Tel: (0800) 169 9169 (freephone)

Relate
Tel: (0845) 456 1310 *(for your local office)*

Relate Direct (counselling by phone)
Appointment Booking Line:
(0845) 130 4016
Email: enquiries@relate.org.uk
Website: www.relate.org.uk

School of Meditation
158 Holland Park Avenue
London W11 4UH
Tel: 020-7603 6116
Website:
www.schoolofmeditation.org

Society of Homeopaths
11 Brookfield
Duncan Close
Moulton Park
Northampton NN3 6WL
Tel: (0845) 450 6611
Fax: (0845) 450 6622
Email: info@homeopathy-soh.org
Website: www.homeopathy-soh.org

Transcendental Meditation
TM-NCO
Beacon House
1–3 Willow Walk
Skelmersdale
Lancashire WN8 6UR
Tel: (0870) 514 3733
(10am–5pm Mon to Fri)
Website: www.transcendental-meditation.org.uk

Women's Health Concern
PO Box 2126
Marlow
Buckinghamshire SL7 2RY
Tel: (01628) 483612
Email: counselling@womens-health-concern.org
Website: www.womens-health-concern.org

Index

Page numbers in *italics* indicate where there are illustrations.